THE
LIVER
CAUSES
HEART ATTACKS

by W.P.Neufeld M.D.

JANIAK

THE
LIVER
CAUSES
HEART ATTACKS

by W.P. Neufeld M.D.

The liver insulted by food ends life suddenly with heart attacks and strokes. Prevention — a scientific explanation...

© 1987
by W.P. Neufeld, M.D.

ISBN No. 0-88925-816-3

Copyright in U.S.A.   1986   TXU261-824
Copyright in Canada   1987   356723

Printed in Canada
Morning Dawn Publishing Company
Box 1158
Surrey, B.C.
V3S 4P6

INDEX

INTRODUCTION

Tom and Mary Lewis were looking forward to dining out that evening, and celebrating their tenth wedding anniversary with friends. After dinner they were to attend a concert together. It was a delightful roast beef dinner they all enjoyed. The meal finished, they were engaged in easy conversation. Suddenly, Tom Lewis turned ashen grey and fell forward with his head striking the table. His shocked wife and friends tried to rest him in a horizontal position on the floor. He was still breathing. An ambulance was called to the scene, and Mary accompanied her husband to the hospital. During the trip, oxygen was administered by the attendant. Meanwhile, preparations were made to receive Tom at the emergency department.

As soon as he arrived, special resuscitative efforts were begun by the hospital staff. After about an hour, a doctor came to tell Mary that all efforts to revive Tom had failed, and that he had died without regaining consciousness.

Tom Lewis was only 42 years of age, a high school history teacher, and the father of three. He was careful about his weight, went jogging regularly, and by all outward appearances was in good health. His death was found to be due to an acute myocardial infarction (heart attack), a shock to the entire community. More than two thousand such tragedies occur in this continent daily. In the United States alone, over one million coronary attacks take place every year, of which some 540,000 are fatal. Another 170,000 lives each year are claimed by strokes.

In my fifty years as a medical practitioner, I have treated thousands of medical cases, and have observed that many occurrences of heart attack and stroke have followed a typical American meal, similar to the one consumed by Tom Lewis. These observations forced me to explore some of the reasons why so many people suffer a heart attack after eating. Which food items, if any, would increase the risks of heart attacks and strokes, and which body organs come into play that can affect the blood circulation, blood pressure and heartbeat? Are the heart and brain the only organs affected, or do other organs within the body affect the heart and circulatory system? Can we view adverse organ reactions as isolated occurrences, or could they be the result of a chain reaction, where one organ can affect the others?

Speaking as a physician, I feel that the factors which can contribute to heart attack and stroke are extremely important to understand. Both diseases have reached epidemic proportions in the industrialized world, and affect the lives of millions each year.

Despite their frequent occurrence, two-thirds of all sudden heart deaths reveal no history of heart disease. The prime cause of heart disease is atherosclerosis. It is often concealed when the victim is at rest, and can sometimes be detected with an ordinary electrocardiogram.

Medical scientists agree that an unrestricted meat and fat-oriented diet causes atherosclerosis; a disease involving the gradual narrowing of the main arteries of the heart and brain. This arterial degeneration increases more rapidly with obesity, smoking, diabetes, and a sedentary lifestyle.

Along with the gradual development of atherosclerosis, we would expect a corresponding deterioration of the mind, and the progressive weakening of the body as a whole; with ample warnings of an impending heart attack or stroke. However, this is sometimes not the case. There may be no warning symptoms whatsoever. The victim may suffer the sudden attack while chatting with friends, watching television, or enjoying an afternoon nap. The "how and why" of the sudden heart attack and stroke is still baffling to most physicians and medical researchers, despite many years of study and clinical observation.

As the central organ of the body, the liver is composed of some 350 billion cells. They are not only responsible for nourishing every cell in our body, but also break up, detoxify and destroy any harmful chemicals which enter the body through the mouth, skin and lungs. When this highly complex organ is bombarded daily by harmful foods, a marked derangement of its cells can result. With each allergic disturbance, the liver cells swell up with water, and can suddenly change their normal metabolic function to an obstructive dysfunction. It is with this allergic reaction of the liver cells that the liver obstructs the flow of the

9

blood towards the heart. Consequently, such a major liver disturbance can set the stage for a serious crisis, such as a heart attack or cerebral vascular **thrombosis** (stroke).

Based on my own experience in medicine and the epidemiological studies I have pursued in regard to this problem, I am convinced that the **acquired allergic reaction of the liver**, to certain foods, (especially **denatured** meat and animal fat) is the primary cause of sudden heart attacks and strokes. I also found that a carefully selected vegetarian-style diet cannot only prevent a heart attack but also help regenerate the liver after an allergic reaction and help in the prevention of premature sudden death from these and other diseases.

In the following chapters, we will explore the basic structure and functions of the liver, heart and brain, and document how an allergic liver reaction to certain foods can lead to a sudden heart attack, stroke, and other physical disorders. Special attention will be given to the unique role of the liver as the body's central organ, and how a healthy, strong liver can benefit the entire body.

This book will also examine the importance of a proper diet in maintaining a healthy liver. We will offer dietary recommendations, that will provide sound nutrition while helping us to reduce the risk of heart disease, stroke, and other degenerative diseases. Finally, we will explore how regular exercise can help regenerate a damaged liver, the heart and the circulatory system, and keep our bodies strong and healthy.

Sudden heart deaths and strokes **can** be prevented.

I am convinced that only when we begin to understand the liver, and the vital role it plays in health and disease, can we achieve a level of optimum health, and realize our full potential as human beings.

ABSTRACT

Much has been written about how the coronary and cerebrovascular atherosclerosis reduces myocardial or cerebral function and how it increases the risk of myocardial and cerebral infarction. The cardiologists and pathologists describe in detail the arterial disease, but are still seeking the cause of "the sudden event" that leads to an acute myocardial or cerebral infarction. A new concept is presented regarding the cause of these vascular accidents. It is conceivable that the anaphylactic reaction of the liver causes these catastrophic events to occur. The experimental evidences and clinical observations are presented. The liver has a strangulating control of the blood circulation when insulted by improper food. With an anaphylactic reaction the return venous blood flow to the heart is blocked by the liver. At the same time the coagulative components of the blood are increased causing myocardial or cerebral infarctions.

Heart attacks and strokes abruptly terminate almost one million lives each year on the North American continent.

The public is helplessly waiting for medical scientists to stem this massive slaughter. This scourge of the twentieth century — this "sudden event" blights or

13

ends many active, useful lives below the age of sixty-five... needlessly.

The urgency of the problem is obvious, for myocardial infarction strikes some victim every twenty seconds. It is imperative, therefore, that every possible cause and every possible solution be intensively examined without prejudice. *(1-12)*

The anaphylactic reaction of the liver should definitely be considered as the cause of this great and unnecessary killer. This anaphylactic reaction was clearly documented at the beginning of the twentieth century but studiously ignored by modern medicine. It should now be recognized as the leading reason for most myocardial and cerebral infarctions.

The possibility that an insulted liver insidiously strangles the heart and brain should motivate every allergist to the most careful study of this phenomenon.

We shall now present the hypothesis in more detail.

It is possible that the sudden heart deaths that complicate coronary atherosclerosis are caused by an anaphylactic reaction of the liver cells, due to food or any substance that the cells are sensitized to. By such a reaction the return flow of blood in the Portal vein, the Hepatic artery and in some instances the Inferior Vena Cava to the heart is impeded by the swollen congested liver. With this reaction is associated a drop in blood pressure, a decrease in cardiac output, a hemoconcentration and an increase of the blood coagulation components. *(4)*

The sudden change in the hemodynamics causes the ischemia of the heart muscle and conducting mechanism, especially when the blood in its viscid condition at lowered pressure, meets a stenotic coronary artery. *(5)* All varieties of cardiac arrhythmias, including fibrillation, all varieties of vascular myocardial damage from focal or diffuse subendocardial coagulative myocytolysis to transmural coagulative necrosis are simply due to ischemia, dependant in part or altogether on the intensity and length of the anaphylactic reaction of the liver.

To the casual observer, the liver, motionless and dull colored is one of the least impressive organs of the body. It weighs 1500 grams and is comprised of about 1,000,000 lobules each of which hold 350,000 cells. *(13)* The blood perfuses these many cells as it flows through the sinusoids. Because of its enormous metabolic activity the liver requires 1500 cc of oxygenated blood every minute. This is 25 percent of the total circulation, while it carries about 20 percent of the total oxygen required by the body. *(14)*

Two main vessels supply the liver with nutrients, the Portal vein and the Hepatic artery. The blood from these two vessels joins before it flows through the millions of microscopic canals called sinusoids. The sinusoidal canals are lined on either side with liver cells where the blood comes in immediate contact with the cells and the exchange of metabolites, the nutrients from the digestive system, takes place. Furthermore, the sinusoids are provided with inlet and outlet sphincters under nerve control, which regulate the flow of blood through the liver. *(13)* They are under both sympathetic and vagal influence. The response to Ephedrine is dose dependant, causing constriction of sinusoidal sphincters within ten to thirty minutes. *(15-18)* The practical mechanism of the sinusoidal canals has been well documented. They close when the sensitized liver cells, which line the sinusoids, react by swelling to any foreign substance or food in the blood as it flows through the canals. Furthermore, the sinusoidal canals are also closed when the sphincters, located on each end of the canals, contract in response to sympathetic nerve stimulation. *(19-22)*

The Anaphylactic Reaction

The word anaphylaxis (ana- against, phylaxis- protection) is defined in Dorland's Illustrated Medical Dictionary, "as an unusual or exaggerated allergic reaction of an organism to foreign proteins or other substances." Anaphylaxis is an antigen-antibody reaction. The term was originally used to describe an allergic reaction of liver cells which had been sensitized in laboratory animals by injecting a foreign substance such as horse serum. The terms called hypersensitivity, immune reaction or foreign protein reaction are also used to describe anaphylaxis. This knowledge has since been extended to human reaction as well. *(3-5)* Any injection or ingestion of a foreign substance can render some individuals hypersensitive to that same substance at a later date.

The name and concept of anaphylaxis was born at the beginning of this century. *(10)* It was diligently pursued by various investigators for about 30 years. Since then the original work of these scientists has been repeatedly confirmed. The electron-microscope during the last few decades permitted direct visual observation of this impressive phenomenon, so that this branch

16

of human physiology could be well documented. *(23-65)*

It is the prevailing opinion that an anaphylactic reaction is always violent, and even fatal. When in fact allergic, immune, anaphylactic or foreign protein reactions vary considerably. Some can be fatal or mild, depending on the antibody buildup and how much antigen has entered the body by injection or ingestion. Such reactions are often associated with a disturbed blood circulation. A strong reaction may lead to irreversible shock whereas a minor circulatory disturbance due to anaphylaxis, may pass with a fleeting spell of "lightheadedness" due to hypotension. Allergists also agree that in an acute anaphylactic shock up to sixty-six percent of the blood volume can be held out of circulation by the liver. *(55)*

It is easy to understand why most sudden heart deaths do not occur after an acute exertion, but at rest, either sitting in a chair, resting on a couch or in bed. *(49)* When a person is inactive or has a sedentary occupation the blood (especially after a heavy meal to which he is sensitive) shifts more from the extremities into the splanchnic pool. When an anaphylactic reaction of the liver takes place this volume of blood is trapped in the abdomen. This in turn reduces the venous blood flow to the heart more suddenly than if the victim were active and on his feet. If the anaphylactic reaction occurs while he is moderately active the extremities require a greater portion of the five thousand cubic centimeters of blood that is available in an adult. Hence, during an anaphylactic reaction the liver can only trap a smaller volume in the splanchnic pool while the blood from the extremities and trunk is available and free to return to the heart unhindered to sustain the coronary perfusion during the critical moments of the reaction. If the coronary vessels were free of atherosclerosis it would take an unusual strong reaction to cause an acute ischemic coagulative myocytolysis or an ischemia of the conducting mechanism to result in a cardiac arrest. While with advanced coronary atherosclerosis such an immune reaction need only to be moderate in strength and still cause a transmural myocardial infarction with fatal ending.

Anaesthetic Deaths

An example of cardiac arrest with perfectly normal coronary vessels would be the anaesthetic or recovery room heart death, where at times even adolescent patients succumb. In such instances the victims liver might have been sensitive to the anaesthetic or any drug used in that immediate pre or post-operative period to which the liver reacts anaphylactically. With such a reaction the sinusoids of the liver close and block the return flow of blood from the splanchnic pool. Finally the increased weight (up to fifty percent) of the liver during the reaction could further compress the Cava against the firm muscular and bony posterior wall. The then reduced volume which reaches the heart may be insufficient to sustain the perfusion and viability of the conducting mechanism and cardiac arrest follows. Once this hypothesis has been accepted, the anaesthetic department will prevent such deaths by monitoring the patients sensitivity to drugs and anaesthetic before the operation. Such fatalities will then not occur.

Sudden Death Associated with Heavy Exertion

The history of some patients indicate that the acute myocardial infarction was precipitated by an unusual physical exertion. The cause of an infarction is always myocardial ischemia. The ischemia may be due to an occlusive coronary thrombosis or hypovolemia and associated acute hypotension caused by an anaphylactic reaction. With an anaphylactic reaction of the liver to a meal, "central damage" of the liver lobule due to hypoxia, is always possible. During the time of recovery of this central portion of the lobule (which may take days or weeks) there will be some impediment to the venous return flow through the liver to the heart. A moderate splanchnic pool can develop which may last for days. This reduces the total circulating blood volume available. If such a person suddenly exerts himself physically, the muscles of the body demand extra blood. As the capillaries dilate to supply this need of the extremities the total blood volume can be critically reduced to the embarrassment of the myocardium (Heart). Especially with advanced coronary atherosclerotic narrowing, an acute micro-circulatory collapse with infarction can occur.

Cardiac Irregularities — Arrhythmias

It is usually accepted that cardiac arrhythmias appear when the A.V. or S.A. Nodes or the conducting mechanism have suffered ischemic damage. The extra systoles may appear gradually as we would expect with gradually increasing coronary atherosclerosis. It is also possible that a patient after a heavy dinner goes to bed with a normal cardiac rhythm and wakens in the morning with acute fibrillation. Such heart injury may follow an anaphylactic reaction of the liver to the meal of the night before. The reaction reduces the venous return to the heart causing ischemic damage to the nodes and conducting mechanism. Such conducting injury may be temporary or permanent. Temporary if the injury is slight, healing will follow with improved coronary blood perfusion. On the other hand, if the liver suffers repeated anaphylactic insults, such arrhythmias can become chronically established and require special medical and dietetic treatment.

As we noted, the liver cell can react anaphylactically to any foreign substance but, denatured meat of any kind causes the most common reaction. Food scientists have isolated melonaldehyde, a chemical which appears in all meats by oxidation after it has been cooked and allowed to stand exposed to air even in a refrigerated atmosphere. Melonaldehyde is a breakdown product of unsaturated fatty acids. The longer meat is allowed to oxidize the more melonaldehyde can be extracted. It is possible that patients become sensitized to this chemical and the liver cell reacts anaphylactically. So we find the longer cooked meat is stored before it is served and eaten, the stronger will be the anaphylactic reaction of the liver that has been sensitized.

The science of immunology has progressed steadily since the beginning of this century. Clinicians have been interested in pollens, dusts, molds, spores, animal danders, drugs and food. Besides a thorough history the allergists detect the sensitivity by various immunological techniques. The treatment involves avoiding the antigen and desensitization. In all this work they have a relatively few specific sensitivities of the patient in mind which they discover and treat.

The anaphylactic reaction which aroused the interest of scientists during the early part of this century has almost been forgotten. It is now associated with the rare catastrophic shock reaction due to a drug or insect bite. Not realizing that if there is a strong, sometimes fatal, anaphylactic reaction there must be countless degrees of less severe minor reactions. Since all allergic reactions vary in intensity. Anaphylaxis of the liver is an established law of human physiology and cannot be ignored. The modern concept of allergy discovers that only the exceptional few are affected, whereas anaphylaxis of the liver is a problem everyone experiences. Heart burn, flatulence and abdominal cramps may all be due to temporary portal stasis with hypoxia of the gastrointestinal tract and associated dysfunction.

To point out the difference between the anaphylactic reaction and the modern concept of allergy please note, in allergy only some patients develop a sensitivity and these are found by special examinations when they react to special tests:

— In anaphylaxis **all** animals without exception, that were used for the experiments, reacted as expected.

— In irreversible haemorrhagic shock (one form of anaphylaxis of the liver) **all** ended fatally to the same conditions.

— Traumatic shock (a form of anaphylaxis of the liver) involves **every** victim in similar conditions.

— **All** severe burn cases succumb to an irreversible shock, provided the severity and extent of the injury are the same **due to anaphylaxis of the liver.**

All patients subjected to organ transplants are expected to react with varying degrees of rejection. This is considered to be on an immunological basis. The science of anaphylaxis of the liver involves everyone in contrast to an allergic reaction which affects relatively few.

CHAPTER ONE

THE LIVER

To the casual observer, the liver is one of the least impressive organs of the body. Dark reddish in color and triangular in shape, it weighs approximately 1500 grams (as opposed to the heart, which weighs only 300 grams).

Strategically located in the middle of the body, the liver fits snugly into the undersurface of the diaphragm, connected to it by strong ligaments. This unique relation to the diaphragm creates a suction force which holds the liver in a suspended position. This special suction force can withstand a pull of over forty pounds. The pumping action of the liver/diaphragm movement assists in the circulation of blood through the liver and into the heart. This will be discussed more in detail later on.

In earlier civilizations, the liver was held in the highest esteem. There was a general belief that the liver was at the center of things. No other organ can hold as much blood, nor can perform (with the exception of the brain) so many tasks. Since life and blood were held synonymous by the Babylonians and the Greeks, the liver was considered the central organ of the body and the seat of the human soul.

Despite its rather innocuous appearance, the liver is

clearly the most chemically active "factory" of the body. In order for it to perform its tasks of processing the nutrients for other body tissues and cleansing the body of foreign substances, its structure is both complex and highly sensitized.

The substance of the liver itself is composed of approximately 100,000 tiny lobules similar in size to a grain of millet, measuring about 1/20 of an inch (1 mm) in diameter. In turn, these tiny lobules are composed of numerous Hepatic (liver) cells, each measuring about 1/1000 of an inch (0.025 mm) in size. *(13)* All in all, the liver consists of 350 billion of these specialized Hepatic cells, each of which is responsible for numerous operations vital to our survival.

If we would consider the body as a nation, the liver could be seen as its port of entry, and at the same time, the capital city. The primary function of the liver cells is to assimilate and store those products of food that have been digested by the gastrointestinal system. Some of these digestive products are stored in the liver, while others undergo further processing, preparing them for the use of the body. Their next function is to detoxify any substance which enters the body, or which has accumulated in the body through metabolic processes. The liver cells are also responsible for the secretion of bile. This flows through the gall bladder and bile duct (tube) into the intestine to aid in the digestive process of fats. Furthermore, the liver is the major storehouse of carbohydrates (glucose), proteins, fats, vitamins, and minerals. The 350 billion cells perform their specialized tasks in complete harmony, making the liver among the most important and fascinating of all the body organs.

Despite the intricate functions it performs, the liver itself is soft and pliable, especially when compared to muscle tissue. Liver tissue is almost as soft as brain substance, but it does not enjoy the bony protection of the skull. For this reason, it is highly susceptible to trauma, and although the ribs provide some protection, the liver is easily bruised, contused, or even lacerated.

The Liver and Blood Circulation

Few of us appreciate the enormous amount of oxygen required by these 350 billion liver cells as they perform the vital task of metabolic activity. Each liver cell has many intricate chemical processes to perform, and if the formulae were written, they would easily fill a school blackboard. These processes of purification and nourishment require a continuous supply of oxygen in order to keep the body in optimum health under a wide variety of circumstances.

Unlike the lungs, which receive oxygen through the windpipe, the liver obtains its oxygen through the bood. For this reason it requires a supply of 1-1/2 quarts (1500 cc) of oxygen-rich blood every minute, to profuse it every moment of our lives. *(14)* No other organ of the body requires such a large and continuous flow. Although the mass of the liver comprises only three percent of the total body weight of the average adult, it requires approximately 28 percent of the total circulating blood volume, and over 20 percent of the total available oxygen at all times.

The two major blood vessels involved with the liver

25

function are the **Portal Vein** and the **Hepatic Artery.***
The Portal Vein channels the blood from the stomach,
intestines, pancreas and spleen into the liver, before it
continues onwards toward the heart. This blood is
termed **venous** blood, because it has already partially
given off its oxygen to the digestive tract. It amounts
to about 70 percent of the blood entering the liver.

The Hepatic Artery supplies the other 30 percent of
the liver's blood supply, which is saturated with oxygen and comes to the liver through arteries from the
heart. Within the liver, the blood from these two channels mix and disperses into tiny venules (veins) which
in turn transport the blood into microscopic canals called **sinusoids**. These sinusoidal canals are lined on either
side with liver cells, and bring the blood into immediate
contact with these cells where the exchange of
metabolites (the nutrients from the digestive system)
takes place. We might compare this unit of the liver
to the loading and unloading platform of a factory.
These sinusoidal canals are equipped with a closing or
sphincter muscle at either end, which can either open
to allow the free flow of blood, or close, in order to
contain it, and so obstruct the flow. *(14-18)* This
singular mechanism of the liver provides it with a major control over the general blood circulation. In the
following chapter, we will explore the importance of
this mechanism, and how it can endanger the survival
of the entire body. The contraction of these microscopic
sphincter muscles of the sinusoids can literally determine whether we live or die. *(19-22)*

---

* Remember that arteries channel blood from the heart, while veins carry blood
  towards the heart.

When we consider the role of the liver in general blood circulation, we should be aware of the fact that blood passes through the liver at a very low pressure. When the normal arterial blood pressure is 120 mm Hg. and when the blood leaves the liver through the Hepatic Vein, the pressure is reduced 1 mm Hg. Physiologists state, that it is the pumping movement of the diaphragm, which draws the blood out of the liver into the general circulation. Normally, the body is able to meet the high energy requirements of the liver with sufficient blood and oxygen. However, if the blood pressure drops to a lower level for some reason or other, the cells of the liver may suffer injury by **hypoxia**, a term meaning "not enough oxygen".

Anemia (iron deficiency) also affects the liver cells, which require both normal blood pressure and iron content for their optimum function. The normal iron content of the red blood cells is necessary in order to carry the full capacity of oxygen. In the following chapter, we will explore those conditions which impair the normal functioning of the liver and can lead to a variety of symptoms, some of which can be fatal. However, many of the factors which cause liver malfunction, are under our conscious control, and their understanding can be a determining factor in our own health and that of our loved ones.

CHAPTER TWO

ANAPHYLACTIC REACTION
OF THE LIVER

During the past two decades, the study of immunology (allergies) has moved to the forefront of medical research. In the following pages we will briefly discuss the basics of allergic reactions and explore the role of the liver in this important disorder. Such terms as **immunology, anaphylaxis, allergy,** and **foreign protein reactions** involve similar principles of physiology and will be used interchangeably in this and the following chapters.

Generally speaking, an allergic reaction is simple to understand. When allergy occurs, some cells of the body become sensitized to certain substances called **antigens**, which are introduced from either inside or outside the body. When on a subsequent occasion, the same type of antigen (like pollen) enters the body, it can cause a moderate gradual reaction. Other antigens — such as certain drugs or foreign substances — can produce a sudden more violent reaction. This chapter will deal with the core of this volume — the allergic reaction of the liver cell — because all functions of the liver are affected by this principle. If this essential concept is understood and carefully observed, all other functions of the liver will improve to optimum capacity, with better general health and extended life span.

The Allergic Reaction: What Happens?

When there is an allergic reaction of certain tissues, such as the lining of the nose, the skin or the bronchial tubes, the reacting cells swell up with water. We see this in nasal allergy such as hay fever. The lining of the nose will swell up with water when exposed to an antigen such as pollen from flowers or weeds. This makes breathing difficult.

A similar reaction occurs when the skin is exposed to poison ivy. The welts of the skin that appear when we touch the ivy (antigen) demonstrate the swelling of skin with water. The skin thickens and becomes reddish in color.

A spasm of the bronchial tube causes an attack of asthma when they are in contact with an antigen like pollen. In addition to bronchial muscle spasm, there may be some swelling of the mucosa with water, making breathing difficult.

As in all these instances where the allergically reacting cells swell up with water, so do the liver cells when they react allergically. The digested food molecules are carried by the blood in the Portal Vein to the liver, where they come into immediate contact with the liver cells. As soon as this happens, the reacting liver cells swell up with water. This causes the whole liver to enlarge. It has been demonstrated that during an allergic reaction, the liver increases in weight up to 50% above normal. In other words, a normal adult liver weighing 1500 grams will increase in weight up to 2250 grams. There is one fundamental law of the physiology of the human body: In an allergic or anaphylactic reaction, the cell involved swells up with water. It is the same whether the cell is of the nose lining, the skin or the liver.

The Anaphylactic Reaction

The word **Anaphylaxis** (**ana-** against, **phylaxis-** protection) is defined in **Dorland's Illustrated Medical Dictionary** as an "unusual or exaggerated allergic reaction of an organism to foreign proteins or other substances." The use of the term was originally restricted to a condition of sensitization in laboratory animals, produced by the injection of a foreign substance such as horse serum. This knowledge has since been extended to human allergic reactions as well. The ingestion of a foreign substance, whether taken by injection or through the mouth, can render the individual hypersensitive to the substance in the future. Anaphylaxis is an antigen-antibody reaction. It is also called **hypersensitization, hypersusceptibility** and **protein sensitization**.

The outstanding original researchers in this field were Carl Voeglin, Richard Weil, W. H. Manwaring and J. P. Simonds. Every one of these scientists, with their staff assistance, performed many experiments on guinea pigs, rabbits and dogs. These were then reported in various scientific journals.

A typical experiment to study anaphylaxis was reported as follows: A dog was given a subcutaneous injection of 5 cc of horse serum. Two weeks later it received a large dose of 20 cc of horse serum, intravenously. After this injection the dog immediately went into acute anaphylactic shock. It began to vomit, and had repeated bowel evacuations. Within five minutes the animal began to stagger. This was followed ten minutes later by a period of collapse, associated with a marked drop in blood pressure, so the Carotid pulse (the artery in the neck) could not be felt. The dog died within 30 to 60 minutes after the injection of 20 cc of horse serum, in an anaphylactic shock. Various studies were made to find the exact nature and cause of this acute anaphylactic reaction. The investigators ruled out direct toxicity that might have poisoned the animal. They ruled out heart failure. The sudden dilation of the small capillaries of the whole body were also found not to be the cause of anaphylactic shock. The final documented conclusion, reached after many experiments by various authors, pointed to the liver as the main target of an anaphylactic reaction, with the devastating effect on the whole body, including general vascular dilation.

Abdominal Organs and Anaphylactic Shock

A typical post-mortem report of such an animal was as follows: ''The condition of the liver dominates the pathological impression and presents a picture such as is rarely, if ever, seen under any circumstances. The organ is tremendously swollen. The color is intensely cyanotic (dark red, without oxygen). On section, the cut surface bleeds freely. The Portal Vein (draining the stomach, intestines, pancreas, and spleen) and the Inferior Cava (draining the lower abdomen and legs) are found much enlarged with blood.'' The description of the rest of the digestive organs goes on as follows: ''The gastrointestinal tract may become the seat of severe congestion. There is bleeding into the wall of the stomach and intestine with haemorrhagic (bloody) diarrhea. The pancreas may show some increased swelling. The spleen is markedly enlarged. All this is the result of the Portal blood flow obstruction. The blood meets much resistance to flow in the millions of narrowed sinusoidal canals due to the swollen liver cells in them."

The Mechanism of the Anaphylactic Reaction

Exactly how does an anaphylactic reaction occur in humans, and what process comes into play? In a previous chapter we discussed how the liver works under normal conditions. In order to nourish and purify the liver, this organ requires a steady flow of blood from the heart (via the Hepatic Artery) and from the intestines (via the Portal Vein). Once inside the liver, the oxygen-rich blood from these two channels combines. It then disperses into smaller veins that lead into millions of microscopic canals, called sinusoids.

As stated earlier, the sinusoidal canals are lined with liver cells which come in immediate contact with the flowing blood. When this blood is free from poisons and other toxic materials, the sphincter (closing) muscles at either end of the sinusoid remain open. This permits the liver cells to receive the digested products from the stomach and intestine, and continue on its unobstructed flow towards the Hepatic Vein (the last vein leaving the liver towards the heart) carrying it further toward the heart before being pumped onwards through the body. However, if some foreign substance like denatured protein, a toxin, or other chemical enters

33

the liver to which the liver cells have previously been sensitized, they react allergically. They quickly swell up with water, the sinusoids close down, and the blood flow within the liver and to the heart is impeded. How does this take place?

First of all, it is important to remember that even under normal conditions the blood moves through the liver at a very low pressure. Still there is no difficulty, and 1500 cc (1-1/2 quarts) move through the liver every minute. However, when the liver cells swell up, the sinusoids become narrow and the blood has greater difficulty moving. This obstruction of the blood flow in the sinusoids causes all the liver cells to suffer from lack of oxygen, known as hypoxia. Those cells furthest away from where the fresh blood enters the liver suffer first. The cells expect a fresh supply of oxygen, which is not forthcoming. One by one they are damaged or begin to die from oxygen starvation, which is also known as **necrosis**. Because these dying cells are located in the center of a lobule (a small unit of the liver), the process is called **central necrosis**. It is a very common post-mortem finding by pathologists when performing a post-mortem.

Detail of Central Necrosis

During an anaphylactic reaction, the blood which enters the liver and sinusoidal canals carries a supply of oxygen. After moving through the narrowed canals with great difficulty, only those cells closest to the entrance are getting the needed oxygen. As a consequence, the cells which are located near the center of a lobule are not getting the oxygen they would normally receive, therefore, suffer the earliest injury. If the reaction is strong and long, these cells at the center of the lobule die and wash into the blood. Under such circumstances, central necrosis has occurred.

Over the years, scientists have undertaken numerous studies on liver cell damage due to anaphylaxis, mostly utilizing laboratory animals. One such study was carried out by Dr. R. D. Seneviratne of the University College Medical School in London, involving 98 frogs, 48 mice and 112 rats. The animals were anaesthetized, their abdomens opened, and their liver blood circulation observed through a microscope under a quartz light especially designed for the experiments. Dr. Seneviratne was able to demonstrate how speedily the sinusoids could close and open under various stimuli. This indicated that they were under nerve control. His report contained the following basic findings:

A. Normal blood flow of the liver: "An arresting picture of vivid colors and rapid movement is seen. The blood flow (in the sinusoids) is normally smooth and continuous."

B. After injecting carbon tetrachloride in rats: "Showed centrilobular (central) damage in the liver cells." (Due to hypoxia).

C. Injecting urea (an animal protein): "There was constriction of the sinusoids (with injection into the Portal Vein of 50% of urea), the reaction was almost violent. This was followed by a dilation of the sinusoids lasting three hours." (Effect of hypoxia).

D. After forcing them to breathe nitrogen with

low oxygen tension: "Low oxygen tension in the inspired air results in a dilation (widening) of the sinusoids (filling them with blood). After an hour (the sinusoids) appear to be permanently damaged and remain dilated." (Also due to hypoxia).

E. Under anaesthesia, one limb was crushed of a rat: "There was an immediate marked narrowing of the sinusoids. (The liver cells were swelling up to cause the narrowing of the sinusoid canals). The quantity of blood passing through the liver must necessarily have been reduced. In one hour the sinusoids were packed with red blood cells, not moving (stagnant). Slow blood flow continued in a few. The rats died in about 1-1/2 hours."

This is a picture of an anaphylactic reaction of the liver cells to the debris which turns into a foreign denatured muscle protein, liberated from the injured leg. The same reaction occurs in humans. After a severe traumatic injury in which muscles are crushed, the debris from the traumatized muscle is carried by the blood into the liver. In some cases, such a strong anaphylactic reaction of the liver can cause a state of general shock that ends fatally.

F. Effect of Heat: "A test tube containing water at 30°C. (86°F.) was pressed against the chest wall over the liver. This resulted in a slight dilation of the sinusoid canals. Then the temperature of the water was raised to 40°C. (104°F.) and also held against the right low chest wall over the liver. This caused an immediate contraction of the sinusoids all over the liver." (This could be the effect of sphincter spasms of the sinusoids). Warmth causes dilation, higher temperature cause contraction.

G. Effect of Cold: "A test tube containing water at 10°C. (50°F.) was held against the chest wall over the liver. This caused a contraction of all sinusoids, and stayed as long as the cooling was maintained. Both the heat and cold effect disappeared, when the tube with water was removed from the chest wall. The sinusoids returned to normal size." (Again such reflex effect can be explained only as a sphincter spasm of the sinusoids under nerve control).

Whether we are speaking of laboratory animals or human beings, the constriction of the sinusoids during an allergic reaction can be crucial to survival.

When an anaphylactic reaction is due to some foreign protein, the extent of the damage to the liver cells can vary. When a mild reaction occurs, the liver cells, which are located in the center of the lobule, suffer from mild hypoxia and are only slightly damaged. In such a case, the damage to the liver cells is moderate, and their function returns to normal after several days or weeks.

However, when cells suffer a strong allergic reaction to a foreign protein or any toxic substance, a larger area of cells in the center of the lobule can be completely destroyed. These dead cells are washed away by the blood, leaving only the frame structure of the sinusoidal canals. Such liver injury takes months to heal.

With an Anaphylactic Reaction the Blood Tends to Clot

When an anaphylactic reaction takes place, the blood has a sudden increased tendency to clot. The blood cells become more concentrated, which make the blood thick and gluey. This causes it to move with greater difficulty. This event is usually accompanied by a sudden drop in blood pressure to a subnormal level, making it even more difficult for the blood to move, especially in the vessels of the legs, heart and brain if there is already atherosclerosis. In addition, there is an increased flooding of the circulation with Fibrin and Thrombin (chemicals necessary to clot the blood). These chemicals stored in the liver, are now released into the blood in increased concentration. The stage is now set for a serious catastrophy: The blood may clot in the coronary vessels causing a heart attack, or in the vessels of the brain, resulting in a stroke. Such a tragedy can follow an average American meal.

Although allergic reactions of such magnitude are rare, a moderate anaphylactic disturbance is far more common than most people believe. In most cases, it can be linked to the food we eat. How many among us have experienced a short period of heartburn, halitosis (bad breath), gas, abdominal cramps, vomiting, diarrhea, or sudden constipation? Every person alive has experienced these symptoms at one time or another, but few realize that the reacting liver caused most of these results. The average victim seeks to treat his/her symptoms by going to the drugstore, choosing from a variety of medications to get relief, while ignoring the underlying cause of the problem. If a person is conscious of his/her allergic sensitivities, it is possible to determine which food or substance caused the problem. Those who continue to suffer with persistent distress are advised to consult their physician for a thorough examination of the gastrointestinal tract, including the liver and gall bladder.

Which foods are mainly responsible for this problem? Of all foods, denatured meat (meat which has been chopped, cooked, ground, or otherwise altered from its natural state) has been found to cause the most frequent and violent anaphylactic reactions. Why is this the case?

The major reason is that meat is very susceptible to **oxidation**. In their normal state, the meat cells are covered by a membrane, and are therefore less easily exposed to oxygen. When we grind meat or cook it, this protective membrane is broken. Oxygen is then allowed to enter into the cells, and the oxidation process of the meat is sped up. When meat is ground into hamburger and sausage, or otherwise processed through heating, oxidation is especially likely to occur. Very often this process of denaturization of ground meat, which began when the animal was butchered at the slaughterhouse, speeds up when the meat is exposed to air at the meat counter.

Denatured meat (including red meat, poultry and fish) can provoke the strongest immune reaction. Food scientists have shown that oxidation changes meat to a denatured condition with increasing melonaldehyde content, which increases with time exposed to air. The liver cells in some patients may become sensitized to these oxidative products of meat and react when ingested. Any food or foreign substance may cause such an anaphylactic immune reaction, but not nearly as frequent and severe as meat or meat products.

Due to their chemical composition, all meats are subject to oxidation, including fish and fish products, fowl (especially turkey), beef, mutton, and pork (especially ham). Although oxidation usually goes unnoticed by the consumer, sometimes an advanced stage of oxidation can be seen through color changes in the meat. Turkey meat, for example, has a white or light brown color after cooking, but even after several days in the refrigerator, a greyish or even greenish discoloration can be noticed.

Food scientists warn that fish and other seafood such as crabs, clams, oysters, and shrimp are particularly unstable when exposed to air and normal temperatures. While the denaturization of red meat can take a day or two, that of fish and other seafoods can take only a few hours. Although seafood is usually easier to digest than other meats, this type of food must be handled with unusual speed and care in a cool atmosphere in order to ensure safe delivery to the consumer's table. Canning at sea immediately after the fish is caught appears to be helpful in avoiding oxidation.

It should be cautioned that those people whose livers have already developed a hypersensitivity to meat, manifested by functional dyspepsia, should be especially careful, because the processing and distribution of meat in this day and age is often a complicated and time-consuming affair, with many stages involved. By the time the animal is killed, butchered, and the meat placed in cold storage, transported to the warehouse, butchershop or supermarket, cut up for sale, placed on display, purchased, transported home, prepared and finally served, it has often reached an advanced state of oxidation.

Proteins other than meat are also susceptible to oxidation. Other animal proteins, such as milk, eggs and their products (although much less frequently) are also subject to this process, which cannot always be detected through our sense of taste or smell. The best advice is to be sure to obtain these foods in the freshest state possible, and to store such food air sealed in a refrigerator and eat them as soon as possible.

There are also certain meat analogues on the market made of textured vegetable protein, which often have the color, texture and taste of meat. Even though these protein foods come from plant sources (usually soybeans and wheat) they are often heavily processed, and therefore can also be subject to oxidation. Those who consume these canned meat analogues should try to finish them during one meal. Any leftovers should be removed from the can, wrapped tightly in plastic and refrigerated. These precautions will reduce the rate of oxidation, and will help avoid the possibility of adverse anaphylactic liver reaction.

In a technological society such as ours, obtaining food which is free from pesticides, drugs and other toxins is not an easy task. Because all foreign substances are brought to the liver, this organ is especially vulnerable to allergic reactions from elements found in our food supply. The liver may slowly build up hypersensitivity to these substances, which can suddenly culminate in a major anaphylactic reaction with very serious consequences. For this reason, it is very important to try and scrutinize both the amount and variety of foreign substances which find their way into the body in our food supply. While we must also work to eliminate pollutants in the air we breathe and the water we drink, pure food supply is one that can be more easily controlled.

Extra space has been used on the risk of eating food we have become sensitized to. Denatured meat causes the strongest allergic reaction of the liver. Such a reaction, in turn, can cause a heart muscle damage or stroke. I have no experience with absolutely fresh meat, meat that is being prepared to be eaten as soon as the animal has been slaughtered. I am advising regarding the meat at our market.

CHAPTER THREE

THE LIVER AND THE HEART

In order to obtain the necessary oxygen and nourishment they need, all body cells require a steady flow of blood. In simple organisms, this life-giving fluid is easily diffused throughout the body. In more sophisticated being, such as man, a centrally-located pump is needed to transport the blood to even the smallest microscopic arteries in the most remote areas of the body. This pump is the heart.

The human heart is a pear-shaped muscle, approximately the size of a fist. It is the strongest and most durable muscle in the body. In a fifty-year period, it beats two billion times, and pumps over 300,000 tons of blood. The work done by the heart each minute is equivalent to our lifting a 70 pound (30 kg) weight a foot off the ground. It we were to lift such a weight with the arms every minute, even a professional weightlifter would soon be exhausted. However, the heart performs this work continuously day and night, without even a moment's rest. To enable the heart muscle to perform this work at rest, it itself requires about 225 cc of blood per minute. With a strong exertion, this requirement increases to 1100 cc per minute.

The heart is made up of several chambers which collect and distribute the blood to all parts of the body.

This organ then pumps the blood with tremendous force through the larger and smaller arteries. From the arteries, the oxygen-rich blood flows into smaller and smaller blood vessels, until it enters the smallest microscopic vessels called **capillaries**. The wall of the capillary is only one cell thick. This makes it possible for the oxygen and nutrients to reach and supply every cell of the body. Such ingenious systems of blood distribution functions with a constant blood pressure to diffuse the blood throughout the body, without producing any stress on the vessels.

The blood in the body flows in two directions. Pumped by the heart, the blood flows through the arteries to the head, arms, legs and trunk. From there it returns to the heart through the large veins. This cycle goes on continuously, day and night. In order to function efficiently, the heart must have the same volume return from both the upper and lower halves of the body. Any hindrance to this return flow can cause serious problems.

On its return from the lower half of the body (especially the abdomen and legs) the blood is channeled through the liver on its way to the heart. The portal vein carries the return flow from the digestive organs, while the inferior vena cava returns the blood from the lower abdomen and legs. This structural position of the liver as a passage to the return flow of blood to the heart is of strategic importance with regard to the health and life of the body. It indirectly gives the liver a dominating role over the general circulating blood volume. In other words, the liver has the power to reduce or increase the blood volume that the heart requires every moment, and the heart can pump only the volume it receives.

The Liver and Atherosclerosis

Under ideal circumstances, the blood is permitted to flow through the clean arteries and veins without obstructions of any kind. However, those who adopt the normal high meat and high fat diets of the United States, Canada, Western Europe and Australia, experience a build-up of fatty patches in the blood vessels, which is known as **atherosclerosis**. This coating of the arteries obstructs the flow of blood to the heart muscle, and can result in gradual weakening of the heart, or precondition the arteries to an acute heart attack. How does this build-up come about? A major factor is high blood cholesterol. Before developing atherosclerosis, there usually is a high cholesterol blood level, a fat which coats the inner walls of the arteries. Cholesterol is a direct consequence of a high fat and meat diet. Cholesterol is made by the liver from fat.

During the last century, there has been a tremendous increase in the consumption of fatty and cholesterol-rich foods. Meats, eggs, fats, dairy products, fried foods, and rich pastries have achieved enormous popularity in countries such as ours. They are being eaten in far greater amounts than the human body was designed to cope with. When we realize that the normal American, for example, consumes some 700 milligrams of cholesterol a day in food, we can understand the strain the liver is subjected to when it is caused to eliminate the excess cholesterol into the bile.

Once the blood has a high level of cholesterol, which

45

is often joined by high levels of other fats (such as triglycerides and phospolipids), these substances act as a kind of "floating oil", which attaches fatty plaques along the walls of the 80,000 miles (49,600 km) of the body's arterial channels.

As the inner coating of such fat deposits thickens, the channel of the artery becomes narrower and narrower. The most common sites where atherosclerotic deposits are found are the arteries of the heart muscle, the brain, the aorta (the largest artery leading from the heart) and the arteries of the arms and legs. No one knows why these blood vessels are more frequently affected than the others.

When these arteries are clogged, the organs or tissues they supply suffer from a reduced supply of blood, known as **ischemia**. This is more common than many would believe, as we observe the growing number of middle-aged men and women, who once were full of vigor and vitality, begin to slow down prematurely. The cause of this decline in strength can be the narrowed arterial channels that allow only a reduced blood supply to reach the body's tissues. When the coronary vessels of the heart become more narrowed with fatty deposits, shortness of breath and fatique begin to appear sooner, and tend to last longer. Sudden bursts of activity (such as running to catch a bus), begin to cause chest discomfort.

As the arterial narrowing increases, this discomfort becomes more noticeable, and often changes into a definite pain. The heart beats may now become irregular, and the victim begins to refrain from any exertions which will produce a tightness or pain across the chest or left arm.

Unfortunately, this is the story of millions of men and women in our modern Western Society. Once the heart is damaged by **infarction** (when a whole section of the heart muscle dies because of insufficient blood supply), or many of the muscle fibers are scarred due to ischemia (also caused by an insufficient blood supply), the whole body is weakened and partially maimed. With the arteries of the body gradually closing up, the function of the whole body also gradually deteriorates.

The Liver and Sudden Heart Deaths

In the last few pages, we have explored the basic reason how the arteries can get clogged, with the gradual appearance of symptoms that follow. Most friends and relatives can accept the gradual decline in strength of the one they love. What shocks them, however, is the sudden, unexpected heart attack or stroke which was described in the introduction of this book. *(95-98)* Even though the coronary arteries are slowly being narrowed by fatty deposits, the individual may still be able to put in a full day's work, jog regularly, and project the very image of health and vitality. Yet, suddenly, and without warning, this person drops dead of a massive heart attack or stroke. *(99-100)* What causes so many of these mysterious deaths? Based on my forty-five years of clinical experience, with extensive research in the literature regarding this problem, I am fully convinced that the allergic reaction of the liver to some food or substance is the cause of the sudden heart attack or stroke.

As was pointed out earlier, the blood stream flows in two directions. First pumped away from the heart along the arteries towards the head, arms, legs, and abdomen, the blood then returns back to the heart through the three large veins: the portal, the superior, and inferior vena cava (see illustration). In order to pump this blood effectively, the heart must receive a steady full volume return flow from both the upper and lower halves of the body. Normally, there is no difficulty with this return flow. However, there can be a problem with the return flow from the lower half of the body, if it is impeded by the liver. During an allergic (anaphylactic) reaction of the liver, the liver obstructs this return flow, and the heart finds itself short of blood. This produces a sudden ischemia of the heart muscle. In addition, it has been well documented in medical literature that when an anaphylactic reaction of the liver occurs, the blood has an increased tendency to clot. *(71-77)* Hence, in a strong anaphylactic reaction of the liver, there is both a hindrance to the return flow of blood, and a tendency for the blood to clot, which can produce a sudden and often fatal cardiac arrest or stroke. *(111-112)*

Let us take the example of Tom Lewis, an outwardly healthy person who jogs every day. At the age of 40, he was probably unaware of the damage he had already suffered. His coronary arteries, over the years, had developed patches of fat along the walls. The coronary arteries, although narrow at a few points, still allowed him to play golf and run without discomfort. He joined his wife and friends at a dinner party, and had roast beef with all the trimmings. While still eating, he suddenly had acute chest pains, and was rushed to the hospital, where he was pronounced dead.

How is such a disaster possible? The digested meat molecules arrive in the liver, usually in one to three hours. His liver cells had been sensitized to this particular type of roast. His wife and friends, though eating the same food, may not suffer an allergic reaction at this time. In reacting to this protein, the liver cells that line the sinusoids swell up and constrict the sinusoidal canals, thereby obstructing the return flow of blood to the heart. The blood pressure drops. At the same time, the blood becomes thick and gluey. When this occurs, the heart suffers from ischemia. At a point where the arteries have been narrowed by atherosclerosis (usually in the heart or brain), the blood cannot get through due to low blood pressure and the viscidness of the blood. As a consequence, the tissue of the brain or heart muscle beyond this narrow point, receives no blood. *(113-114, 128-129)* If this blockage occurs in a large coronary artery, the heart stops and the victim dies. *(115-116)* If a smaller branch of the coronary artery is involved, a smaller area of the heart muscle dies. In this case, the victim will live, and the damaged part of the heart will heal in time, although a scar can remain for life. If blockage involves an artery of the brain, the person may die or be partially paralyzed. *(122-124)*

I would now like to present as an example, the history of one of my patients who suffered two heart attacks shortly after she consumed meals, which evidently contained denatured meat protein. On May 25th, Mrs. V. was brought into the emergency department by ambulance, seriously ill. She had chest pains radiating down her left arm. She was very pale, and was evidently in shock. A physical examination, electrocardiogram, and laboratory tests confirmed my suspicion that she had an acute heart attack, also known as a **myocardial infarction.** A cardiologist was called in for consultation. He confirmed the diagnosis, and treated Mrs. V. during her hospital stay. A few days after admission, when she was well enough to talk, I asked Mrs. V. what she had eaten for dinner on the night she had the attack. She answered, "Oh, there was some stew left over in the refrigerator, which I had for dinner." She had her dinner at 6:00, and by 8:30 she felt acute chest pain, for which she was admitted to the hospital. Mrs. V. was living alone at the time, and had just finished washing the dishes. There was no undue stress or exertion before the heart attack, nor could she remember any special strain of any kind during the weeks leading to the attack.

Mrs. V. remained in the hospital until June 15th, when she was discharged. I took great care to explain to her the danger of eating denatured meat, that it could upset her liver, and lead to another heart attack. I also advised her to restrict her activity, as she still experienced some chest pain.

On September 19th, Mrs. V. was again admitted to the emergency ward with another attack. The examinations confirmed that she had suffered another infarction of the heart muscles. Mrs. V. admitted that a few hours before the attack, she had eaten cold chicken that was left over from the previous day.

Three hours after the meal, she experienced her chest

50

pains. Fortunately for Mrs. V., this infarction was not as severe as the first one. However, her cardiologist was worried and warned that her next attack may be her last.

The day she was discharged from the hospital, I had a long talk with Mrs. V. and her daughter about the seriousness of her condition, and explained to both the risk she took, every time she ate denatured meat in any form. I advised Mrs. V. to have no red meat, fish, nor fowl, and no meat soups or extracts. She decided to follow this advice. Because the repeated heart attacks considerably reduced Mrs. V.'s strength, I advised her to move into a nursing home. It was agreed that her daughter would take her to her own home, in another city, and care for her. One year later, I enquired about Mrs. V. She was alive and well, and had suffered no further attacks. At this writing, she is healthy, and she continues to adhere to her meat-free diet.

The medical history of Mrs. V. illustrates the close relationship between a meal containing denatured meat and heart attack. It takes about from one to two hours after eating for the food molecules to arrive in the liver (the attacks have also been observed occurring during the night, following the dinner). As soon as these meat molecules come into contact with the liver cells, which have been sensitized to the particular condition of the meat, they swell up. When swollen, these cells restrict the returning blood flow to the heart. With a critically reduced blood flow, because of the liver cell reaction, the heart either stops contracting, or is variably damaged. *(111-116)* Furthermore, a clotting tendency develops during the reaction, and the blood turns viscid. These factors together lead to a decreased blood flow that can cause a thrombosis or clotting in the heart or brain arteries *(123-128)*, especially if there is a narrow point due to atherosclerosis. The heart muscle that is supplied by such an artery dies (infarction). *(116,118)* In the brain, a stroke occurs. *(129-131)* In medical terms: brain infarction, (an artery that supplies blood to certain area of the brain is closed by a clot) that area of the brain dies.

Why Heart Deaths Occur at Night

It is known that most heart attacks occur while the victim is asleep or resting. According to the medical textbook **Diseases of the Heart,** *(117)* "Among 1108 attacks of acute coronary thombosis, 52% occurred while the patient was asleep or resting, 21% during mild routine activity, 16% while the patient was walking, and 9% during moderate activity. In only 2% was there a history of unusual physical exertion."

Such findings could be due to the following reason: Our general blood circulation is arranged in such a way that the local demands for blood, in any part of the body, will be met with an increased volume. For example, a runner needs a greater supply of blood in the legs. During a race, the blood vessels in the leg muscles will dilate, thus increasing the amount of blood flowing to these muscles. The boxer or weightlifter generally requires more blood in the arms. During a workout, the local blood vessels in the arms and legs will dilate, and will permit the flow of oxygen and glucose-rich blood into the arms and legs. When a person lies down to rest, the blood has a tendency to shift from the arms and legs into the blood vessels of the abdomen. This shift is particularly evident after the person lies down after a heavy meal, because the digestive processes require more blood. The enlarging liver, reacting to the meal, obstructs the return flow of blood, and causes the abdominal vessels to dilate and pool the blood there.

Even under normal circumstances, the liver cells swell moderately when the digestive food products are being carried in for processing. However, the cells enlarge much more if they react anaphylactically to food. The liver cells constrict the sinusoidal canals by their enlargement. The blood flow from the abdominal organs to the heart meets this resistance in the liver. A "blood pool build-up" now occurs in the abdominal vessels, making less blood available to the heart and the rest of the body. As expected, the heart will now suffer from a critically reduced return blood flow during this period. With insufficient blood available, the heart stops or is damaged. *(111-118)*

As stated before, when an anaphylactic reaction of the liver takes place, this event becomes more intensified. As the liver cells swell, the sinusoids become blocked. The liver fills up with stagnant blood that does not move, and can enlarge to as much as fifty percent above its normal weight because with such mechanical obstruction, it is difficult for the blood to flow from the digestive organs through the liver, back into the heart. This is why heart attacks are more frequent when a person sleeps or is resting, rather than when he is active. When a person is up and active, the blood is drawn to the extremities. From there, it can return to the heart,

53

unhindered even during an anaphylactic liver crisis, and possibly saves the person's life.

Anatomists and allergists agree that, from fifty to sixty percent of our total blood volume can be locked in the abdominal veins during an anaphylactic liver reaction. When this occurs, the overall blood pressure drops, the blood to the heart becomes thick, and the fibrin (a blood clotting chemical) increases in concentration. This makes the blood gluey, and will clot, or at least not flow through, at the narrowest point of the coronary artery. Consequently, a fatal heart attack can occur. *(116-118)* If a smaller branch of the coronary artery is closed by the clot, the heart muscle beyond the clot will die. *(94)* In this instance, the victim may survive, but a scar will replace the dead muscle area. In the brain, a certain part will die. *(122-125)*

The Liver and Physical Activity

If either a housewife, laborer or clerk suffer an anaphylactic reaction after a meal while they are up and about, they are not as likely to suffer a heart attack, because the blood is not as much confined in the vessels of the abdominal organs as with a person sitting or lying down. During activity, the blood circulation is equally divided between the abdomen and the extremities. The unimpeded return flow from the extremities will provide the heart with the blood during the critical minutes of the reaction. It is this unhindered return flow from the extremities that prevents an ischemic crisis of the heart during an anaphylactic reaction. The more likely victim of such a disaster would be the executive sitting behind the desk at work, or as he rests on a couch in the den after a heavy dinner. When a person is occupied with moderate activity, the circulating blood volume is more evenly divided between the extremities (arms and legs) and the abdomen. If a victim now partakes of a meal to which the liver reacts allergically and soon is moderately active, the consequences to the heart will tend to be less extensive. Because the blood volume is more equally divided between the extremities and the abdomen, the return flow of blood from the arms and legs would supply the heart with a sufficient amount of blood through an anaphylactic crisis. The blood from the extremities, on its return flow, is less impeded by the liver that blocks the return flow from the Portal Vein and its branches. This is also the reason why those who perform physical work to earn their livelihood (such as farming, construction or factory work) are less likely to suffer heart attacks and strokes. However, as soon as they retire from such work, these individuals are exposed to the same danger as the sedentary executives or business people who are prone to suffer these vascular catastrophes. The heavy physical worker tolerated heavy meals during the time he was working, but the risk comes after he retires and continues this habitual heavy diet, with much less physical activity. At this time of life, if the liver is being overloaded with heavy foods, (causing a larger volume of blood to shift into the abdomen), a sudden allergically reacting liver locks the blood in the abdomen, and so critically depriving the heart of blood. *(121)* Because of general inactivity, blood will always tend to congest the abdominal organs of a heavy eater instead of the extremities, as occurred during the more

55

active years.

An example from my medical practice involves Alfred M., a garage mechanic. He enjoyed overall good health, except that he suffered from moderate arthritis in both knees, which sometimes interfered with his work. He had no previous signs or symptoms of heart trouble. On June 7, 1973, he and his wife returned by ferry from an island holiday. While aboard the ferry, he enjoyed a hamburger for lunch. Two hours later, he suffered acute chest pains and vomited. On landing, his wife brought him to the emergency department of the local hospital. After examination, he was found to be the victim of an acute myocardial infarction with a digestive upset. He was referred to the care of a cardiologist. Every effort was made to save his life, but his heart was damaged so badly by the infarction, that he died of congestive failure in two months. This illustrates how an an anaphylactic disturbance of the liver, due to the meat that Mr. Alfred M. had been sensitized to, can lead to a serious heart damage and death.

It was likely that Mr. M. enjoyed his hamburger, and that many others on the ferry undoubtedly had the same lunch and experienced no discomfort. However, Mr. M.'s liver cells were hypersensitive to the specific molecular denaturization of the meat. That the liver reacted allergically was indicated by his simultaneous digestive upset. Vomiting and chest pains appeared at the same time. What happened in this instance is well-documented by medical science.

An observation should be made for those who have a sensitive digestive system. The meat on airplanes, trains and ferries, are sometimes cooked beforehand.

After cooking, it is frozen, packed, and placed aboard the transit unit. When needed, the food is then heated and served. In this process, it is possible that the meat has oxidized during handling. *(150-154)* Freezing, although retards the process, does not prevent such oxidation, and some people may also react allergically to such denatured meat. Of course, many people can eat this denatured meat with no discomfort, and with no apparent allergic reaction. But, the risks are with the hypersensitive. Safety is in prevention. Don't take any chances, especially if you have some digestive problems. There is no doubt in my mind that Mr. M. could have prevented his premature death. In my opinion, had he followed a (meat-free) vegetarian diet, accompanied by regular exercise, he would likely be alive today. The liver is the target of all food reactions, and if the liver cells are sensitized to a certain condition or state of the meat, the allergic reaction that follows can damage the heart fatally.

We have frequently been saddened when our friends or acquaintances suffer a sudden heart attack or stroke soon after their retirement. For this reason, we warn them before they retire that they should get used to a low fat and meat, vegetarian-style diet, and physically remain active under a doctor's supervision. I believe this to be one of the reasons why the wife usually outlives the husband. Although the woman's blood chemistry (with usually lower cholesterol content) is in her favor, I believe the continual physical activity involved in housework is one of the important reasons that she suffers less frequent vascular occlusion (clotting) of the heart or brain arteries. Without a doubt, the idea that the husband should share in the housework is as life saving for him as it is for his wife.

The Liver and Heart Irregularities

Moderate anaphylactic reactions can occur which damage the sensitive nerve mechanism of the heart, but are not serious enough to cause a detectable myocardial infarction or cardiac arrest. Whenever the return flow of blood to the heart is diminished during an anaphylactic reaction of the liver, the heart soon suffers from variable degrees of ischemia. This damages the nerve mechanism of the heart due to oxygen deficiency and various heart irregularities can manifest themselves. *(4a)*

The heart muscle nerve complex is under the control of a nerve center called the **pacemaker** or **S.E. Node.** *(84)* The role of this nerve center is to send regularly spaced impulses to the heart muscle, which respond with regular contractions. If we would compare the human body to a motor, the pacemaker would be the timer. If the pacemaker suffers from hypoxia due to an anaphylactic reaction of the liver, the heartbeat can suddenly become irregular, producing discomfort and weakness. These "skipped beats" may occur once during every three to ten beats. In some cases, the heartbeats are irregular altogether, depending on the degree of damage the pacemaker has suffered. On the other hand, during an anaphylactic reaction, the heartbeat may increase suddenly to 120 - 150 beats per minute (the normal heartbeat is 60 - 70 per minute), or decrease to 40 - 45 beats per minute. Such heart rate disturbances may be due to hypoxia of the muscle-nerve complex of the heart. This is a state of emergency, and a doctor should be consulted for treatment immediately.

Heart defects that a person is born with are relatively rare, and heart infections due to rheumatic fever or bacterial endocarditis (inflammation of the heart lining) are also relatively infrequent. By far, the majority of heart damages are degenerative in nature, and of vascular origin due to deficient blood supply to the heart muscle and valves caused by atherosclerosis. After such deterioration of the coronary arteries with fat deposits followed by one severe anaphylactic reaction of the liver — with a drop in blood pressure, thickening of blood, and increased fibrin — sets everything ready for a fatal massive heart muscle infarction with cardiac arrest. *(94)*

What causes atherosclerosis? Medical authorities agree on overweight, smoking, diabetes, and lack of exercise. Above all, the food that we eat is the deciding factor in heart disease. Diet plays a major role in the normal endurance of the heart, because the diet tends to maintan a normal liver function on which the heart depends. At a time when ischemic heart disease kills more adults than any other disease in this country, we need to radically change our diet in order to stem this epidemic. This means a prudent diet, low in meat and fats, and one that does not cause atherosclerosis or anaphylactic reactions. Such a diet should substantially lower the serum cholesterol in the blood, and will also enable the liver to be restored to normal function. By carefully maintaining normal liver function and avoiding allergic reactions of the liver, the risk of sudden heart attacks can be greatly reduced or prevented altogether.

CHAPTER FOUR

THE BRAIN, LIVER AND STROKE

The fact that the function of the mind was dependant on the health of the liver has been recognized throughout all ages. Hippocrates (460 - 370 B.C.) states, "Those who are mad on account of phlegm are quiet, but those on account of bile are vociferous, vicious and do not keep quiet." Mental disorders due to the liver disease was also appreciated by Celsus (30 A.D.) and by Galen (131 - 200 A.D.) and up to the 18th century this concept was alive and used in treating patients. However, since the beginning of the 18th century, the status of the liver declined from that of a vital organ to a "great, dull bile producer". Only during the last few decades is the medical world gradually waking up to the importance of this important organ and how it determines both personality behavior and overall health of the whole person.

The brain is the organ that coordinates all the body's functions. Even before we are born, it is the brain which mobilizes and guides our body cells so that they will perform their specialized tasks with both precision and unity of purpose. The role of the brain is to make the body more than just a vast collection of cells, organs and tissues, but a living organism which functions as a unified whole.

Unlike the simpler body organs which have several basic tasks to accomplish, the brain is a highly complex structure which guides and controls thousands of body functions. Like a vast switchboard, the brain works through an intricate system of millions of nerves, and is constantly sending and receiving messages to and from the body's 350 trillion cells in order to coordinate all the body's operations. In fact, if an analogy were to be made between the number of nerve connections in the brain and all the connecting lines in a modern telephone system, the brain would achieve more "thought connections" than a vast network carrying all the simultaneous conversations on every telephone in the world.

What kinds of functions are governed by the brain? As the control center of the central nervous system, the brain regulates a complicated network of both voluntary and involuntary operations: heartbeat, balance, temperature, digestion, defense, locomotion, elimination, respiration, and the adaptation to changes in the environment. Without the brain, we would not be able to speak, hear or experience pleasure and pain. We could not remember the past nor make plans for the future. The brain gathers and stores information and impressions from our inner and outer environments, and makes all the decisions regarding what the body needs and does. Without a properly working brain, our ability to experience and function would be limited to that of a vegetable.

In order to perform these highly complex functions, the brain is dependant on oxygen and glucose which must be supplied continuously and in proper amounts.

Oxygen is required to oxidize the energy producing glucose in the same way that oxygen is required to run a gasoline engine. If we have gasoline in the cylinder but no oxygen, it would be impossible to have combustion. And if we have oxygen without glucose (or glucose without oxygen) the process of **metabolism** (the process chemical changes in living cells by which energy is provided for vital processes) cannot take place.

In this respect, the function of the brain is directly dependant on the function of the liver. In the following pages, it will be shown that since the liver controls the circulating blood volume, it is indirectly responsible for the supply of both glucose and oxygen to the brain. In addition, the crystal-clear cerebrospinal fluid that profuses the brain must be free from toxic chemicals, because the more intricate the cell, the more sensitive it is to any foreign substance. For these reasons, it is important to understand how the function of the liver can affect the brain as both a supplier of blood and a detoxifier of impurities, and see how this interplay will determine our state of health and well-being.

In the following pages we shall deal with the deleterious effect of the nutritional deficiencies of the brain and then the deteriorating functions of the mind injured by toxins that contaminate the cerebrospinal fluid, which surrounds and nourishes the brain.

The Liver and Hypoxia of the Brain

Although the brain comprises only 2.2 percent of our total body weight, it requires approximately 20% of the total amount of oxygen available for the whole body. The brain itself is extremely vulnerable to a lack of oxygen and any interruption of its oxygen-rich blood supply can spell disaster. If there is an occlusion to the blood supply for any reason, such as vascular spasm or stroke, unconsciousness can occur in as short a period as ten seconds. The **cortex**, the seat of the intelligence suffers first. Although the victim may recover physically from a temporary lack of oxygen, traumas such as cardiac arrest, near-drowning, stroke and other conditions which cause fairly prolonged periods of hypoxia can cause severe permanent intellectual deficiences, due to damage of the cortex.

There is no provision made in our brain to store oxygen, because oxygen is utilized by the brain cells as soon as it arrives. As we learned in the chapter on anaphylaxis, when even a mild anaphylactic reaction of the liver takes place, the liver enlarges and the blood supply to the heart and brain is reduced due to a decrease in blood pressure (**hypotension**) and blood volume. The most common symptoms of hypotension include cold feet and hands, general fatigue, listlessness, cloudy vision and dizziness. Any one or all of these symptoms may manifest themselves. After a heavy meat-oriented dinner, many people experience this feeling of sluggishness, due to a moderate congestion of the liver with moderately reduced blood pressure, as part of its normal operations. To satisfy this feeling of drowsiness, some people decide to lie down after a heavy meal. Although this may bring more oxygen to the brain (when we lie down the blood flows more easily into the head), they are unaware of the fact that the drowsiness is due to a moderate hypotension.

In stronger anaphylactic reactions, the status of **hypoxia** (or lack of oxygen) in the brain due to hypotension during sleep is more marked and probably affects millions of people every day. The "morning blues" — early morning depression — is often nothing more than the effect of hypotension from the dinner eaten the evening before, which then starved the brain of oxygen during the night.

The Liver and Hypoglycemia of the Brain

Glucose is literally "the fuel of the cells" and is the other principal element required by the brain. Through a miraculous process in nature, each body cell absorbs all the glucose it needs from the blood, and the process of oxidation supplies the cell with energy. The role of the liver in supplying glucose to the cells is extremely important. When the glucose content of the blood is high after the consumption of a carbohydrate-rich meal, the liver will absorb the excess glucose and store it as **glycogen** (from the Greek — "sugar producer"). When the glucose level in the blood is low, the liver will convert the glycogen into glucose and release the precise amount needed, into the bloodstream to maintain a normal blood sugar level. The brain can function somewhat longer without glucose than it can without oxygen. However, if the supply of glucose to the brain is cut off, the victim can fall into a coma within two minutes, with possible fatal results if prolonged.

There are usually two outstanding factors that most frequently depress the function of the brain: hypoxia brought about by hypotension (low blood pressure) and hypoglycemia (low blood sugar). The sugar or glucose requirement of the brain is just as important as oxygen, and its absence can produce critical results. If a fresh supply of glucose to the brain cells is cut off for as short a time as two minutes, all the glucose that is in the brain would be used up and the function of the mind would cease, and sink into a coma. Usually the intellectual part of the brain (the **cortex**) is the first to suffer from both oxygen and glucose deficiency. Should the supply of glucose be renewed after a severe state of hypoglycemia, the victim could be physically alive, but intellectually deficient, in a state we know as a "vegetable existence". Fortunately, those cases where patients have suffered a severe lack of glucose and oxygen are extremely rare. However, the chronic day-to-day symptoms of hypoglycemia have reached epidemic proportions in this country, and are responsible for a wide variety of brain disturbances.

Symptoms of nervousness, irritability and depression can be linked to hypoglycemia. Every mother knows how irritable children can be when they are hungry just before a meal. After eating, they are calmer and happier. Why? Because their blood sugar has been elevated. Have we not noticed that at the beginning of the meal, visitors at the table are inclined to be slightly tense? When the meal is finished an hour later, everyone is more relaxed and the conversation is fluent and easy. Although such symptoms are easily recognized by most of us, I am inclined to believe that even more serious mental disorders — such as **paranoia** and **schizophrenia** — can be linked in many cases to metabolic deficiencies such as chronic hypoxia and hypoglycemia.

In many cases, both of these disorders occur simultaneously as they are both linked to the same underlying cause: the impaired function of the liver. This impairment can be either the reduced flow of blood to the brain cells during a period of hypotension, or can be traced to the damaged liver's inability to store enough glucose to maintain a normal supply to the brain between meals. When we discuss the symptoms of liver dysfunction in the following pages, hypotension, with resulting hypoxia and hypoglycemia, will often be considered together.

Liver and Stroke

What actually happens in our body to cause a stroke? In a previous chapter we discussed how the typical high-fat, high-cholesterol diet consumed in this country results in a higher concentration of serum cholesterol and other fats in the blood. Over a period of time this fat coats the inside walls of the arteries, narrowing the lumen and making the flow of blood difficult. In advanced cases, we described how the arteries, narrowed by atherosclerotic coating, can suddenly become blocked by local blood clotting during an anaphylactic reaction. A clot will completely stop the flow of blood. The part of the brain that was kept alive by the artery before it closed, dies. This dead section is called a stroke (cerebral infarction).

In addition to the atherosclerosis in the arteries of heart muscle and legs, this arterial coating also takes place in the brain. When this occurs, the inside of the arteries becomes rough and narrow, and the blood flows through these narrowed channels with difficulty. Those brain cells which always need an abundant supply of blood will suffer, and since they do not receive all the oxygen and nutrients they require, they may die. The loss of these nerve cells in the brain, is one factor in promoting the aging process. This can lead to a wide variety of symptoms, such as loss of memory, poor orientation, deficient reasoning ability, and poor concentration.

Neurologists today believe that the insidious loss of mental efficiency that occurs in old age — the process we call senility — is a direct result of day-to-day destruction of a few neurons here and there, until the total loss begins to mount up. This is accelerated by narrowing of blood vessels to the brain due to atherosclerosis.

Today researchers would also blame oxygen and glucose starvation as the actual cause of neuron damage and destruction.

There is also abundant evidence which links the narrowing of the blood vessels in the brain to stroke, the third largest cause of death in modern Western society. A stroke follows the breaking or clotting of an artery in the brain. That part of the brain which was nourished by the artery before clotting, dies.

It has been documented many times that during a major anaphylactic reaction of the liver, the blood becomes viscid, the blood pressure drops, and the fibrin concentration (a clotting factor liberated by the damaged liver) is increased in blood circulation. *(71-77)* When this occurs, all conditions are set for a clot to form. And where will it form first? It will form at some narrow part of an artery where an atherosclerotic patch has narrowed the arterial canal. This may occur in the heart or brain. At such point, the thickened blood cannot get through and the flow stops. The area of the brain that should be supplied by this blocked artery dies from oxygen and glucose starvation. *(122-131)*

I shall relate the tragic story of one patient, Mrs. T. L. She was 67 years of age, and had been under medical care for many years. She visited my office periodically, and in my opinion, the cause of her symptoms were almost always related to food allergy. Usually Mrs. T. L. had digestive complaints such as abdominal pain, nausea, vomiting, and intestinal gas. Careful examinations — including x-rays — revealed that the chest, gallbladder, stomach and intestines were normal, and no organic disease could be found. Indigestion due to allergic reaction to food was her only problem.

As usual in such cases, the liver had developed hypersensitivities to certain foods. Whenever Mrs. T. L. ate food which her liver was sensitized to, she endured her painful symptoms that were cited above. In order to relieve her painful indigestion, she was advised to follow a lacto-ovo vegetarian diet with extra fluids for several days. In addition to her diet, medications were also given to repair the damage of the liver and pancreas, which were damaged by the allergic reaction. Generally, in about a week to ten days after one of Mrs. T. L.'s office visits, she would be feeling much better. She stayed on her diet, even though she had to prepare meat dishes for other members of the family. There were times, unfortunately, when she strayed from her vegetarian diet, and such an occasion was on November 11, 1976.

It was on that day there was a family gathering at her daughter's home. The main course for dinner consisted of roast turkey and sausages, both of which Mrs. T. L. had generous amounts. Unfortunately, she soon fell ill after she returned home, suffering with moderate abdominal distress, which continued through the next day. The other members of the family had no digestive disturbances.

The following morning, Mrs. T. L. was found lying helpless on her living room floor. An ambulance brought her to the hospital where I saw her. Mrs. T. L. was able to nod or shake her head when questioned, but otherwise she was completely paralyzed. She had suffered a cerebrovascular thrombosis at the Pons, an area at the base of the brain pass which controls the body muscles. Mrs. T. L. was conscious, but unfortunately, she was paralyzed. A neurologist was called to give Mrs. T. L. the specialized treatment she required. She was being kept alive by intravenous feedings, but in spite of her family's hopes and prayers for some return of muscular control of body movements, there was no improvement. On December 1, 1976, Mrs. T. L. died. There is no doubt in my mind that the tragic death of Mrs. T. L. was the unfortunate result of eating the turkey and sausage meat. The autopsy showed that Mrs. T. L. had suffered a pathologic change of both the liver and the pancreas.

We know that when such a reaction of the liver occurs the blood pressure sinks, causing the blood to thicken. Viscous blood moves more slowly along the small capilliaries. In this critical phase of the reaction, the blood can clot anywhere, and in this instance, a vital center of the brain was the target for the clot formation. In the case of Mrs. T. L., the reaction occurred 39 hours after eating the meal which could still be in the body, causing a later reaction. Such late reactions are not uncommon, and are recognized in the science of immunology. We should remember that Mrs. T. L. experienced abdominal pain very shortly after the meal, which continued through the next day. When we examined her in the emergency department on November 13th, she groaned every time the abdomen over the liver and pancreas was touched.

In the United States alone, an estimated one and a half million people suffer a stroke each year. For both the stroke victims and their families, the tragedy often brings untold suffering and agony from the crippling that often results. Through a proper understanding of the relationship between anaphylactic reactions of the liver and stroke, I believe that much of this needless suffering will be eliminated.

With proper diet and exercise, life can be more enjoyable in spite of advancing years. The degenerative maladies of advancing age, such as high blood pressure, heart attack, stroke, and rheumatism, do not need to cloud our final years. The regular American-style diet invites early invalidism. In contrast, a disciplined lifestyle based on proper foods and regular exercise, is a joy to both our children and grandchildren. An older, healthy person has the benefits of exuberant health, and a vital, active life. With the accumulated wisdom of a lifetime of experience, he or she can be a role model for growing children. Such a person is an asset rather than a burden to the family, and can serve as a true source of stability in these turbulent times.

CHAPTER FIVE

PREVENTION

The Liver and Food

In a broad sense, all substances that enter the body must be pure, clean, non-poisonous, and life-sustaining. The air we breathe should contain the normal pure constituents of oxygen, nitrogen and water, and should be free of any other contamination such as gases, smoke (including tobacco) and dust. Buildings should be well ventilated, to cleanse the atmosphere of gases and chemical dust. The water we drink should be under the surveillance of health inspectors, and be free of chemical or bacterial contamination. The food we eat should be pure, wholesome and nourishing, and contain all the necessary constituents of carbohydrates, proteins, fats, vitamins, and minerals. In the developed countries such as ours, nutritional deficiencies are due more to ignorance than the lack of availability of nutritious food. What cannot be obtained fresh from the garden or orchard, has to be stored or crated for shipping. Here is where the greatest caution should be exercised in order to prevent spoilage by either refrigeration or dehydration.

Allergic Sensitivity

The issue concerning how we can heal a damaged

liver can be divided into two basic areas. The first area involves the method by which we can help heal an already damaged liver, both quickly and effectively, while the second involves those foods that facilitate optimum recovery of liver function and prevent liver cell injury.

In the introduction to this book, we spoke of contaminated and spoiled food which the health department of every city and town is supposed to prevent from reaching the food market and the kitchen of the consumer. However, there is one destructive food disturbance that is far more common and devastating than food contamination and spoilage combined: anaphylactic reaction of the liver to food items to which the liver cells have become sensitized. No health department can inspect and prevent this form of food disturbance. It is a problem to be settled by the patient with the help of a physician. Although the particular food in question may be considered to be clean, nourishing, well-preserved and acceptable by many people, it is rejected by those whose liver cells have become sensitized to it. To them, it is like poison, which can either temporarily paralyze or destroy a great part of their three and one-half billion liver cells. What steps can the victim take to heal the damaged cells and restore them to normal function?

Body Cleansing

During much of our lives, our bodies ingest a wide variety of toxins, which enter the body through swallowing and inhalation. Many of these toxins are removed by the liver and the other organs of elimination. The major toxins (known as endotoxins) are either the end products of body metabolism (in the form of waste) or are formed by the special production of the bacterial activity of the colon. This situation is especially found when the colon is filled with rapidly decaying protein residue from foods such as meat. In the course of their normal metabolic activity, these bacteria produce a toxin when one is constipated.

If the bowels move well once or twice daily, and little or no meat is ingested, the liver can normally detoxify the blood before it enters the general circulation. However, if a person is suffering from a marked liver dysfunction, due to a recent anaphylactic reaction of the liver to food, the liver is unable to destroy and discharge all the toxins that are produced. When the victim is admitted to a hospital vomiting, after careful examination we have found the only cause, that the colon is often constipated. The bacterial toxins from the colon have begun to overwhelm the beleaguered liver, and have entered the general circulation and the brain. This explains the mental confusion and disorientation we sometimes observe when such a disturbance occurs.

When the liver is injured, and normal body metabolism is impaired, a period of fasting is often beneficial to stimulate the body's cleansing mechanism. The best kind of fast that is designed to treat a disturbed liver is a temporary water fast that can be undertaken either at home or (in serious cases) under hospital supervision.

If the patient is admitted to a hospital ward, he/she will be allowed only small sips of water because of the nausea that often accompanies an anaphylactic liver reaction. In such cases, the patient is given intravenous fluids day and night, at an average rate of 100 cc an hour. This kind of "fasting treatment" is continued for 48 - 72 hours, depending on the speed of recovery. If the blood is found to be deficient of any nutritive substance (such as vitamins and minerals) they are added to the intravenous fluid. Glucose is also added to the intravenous fluid so that the patient receives from 100 - 150 grams every twenty-four hours. Glucose supplies some of the calories that are required by the body, and facilitate the normalization of liver function.

When the patient is not ill enough to be hospitalized, a short fast from one to two days (depending on the degree of anaphylactic disturbance) is often advisable. Under the supervision of a medical doctor, a typical fast would involve drinking about 2000 cc (about two quarts) of water or pure fruit or vegetable juice every twenty-four hours taken with liberal amounts of honey, if tolerated. The glucose which the honey provides will help to restore depressed liver function more quickly, while the water "flushes out" many of the toxins that have accumulated in the body.

As the body is being cleansed of foreign protein, chemicals and toxins by ingesting large amounts of fluids, special attention needs to be given to the colon itself, to help free it of all fecal residue. In some cases, the patient will begin cleansing out the body through fasting, while neglecting the toxins that are already impacted within the colon. When the function of the liver is depressed after an anaphylactic reaction, it is not able to disintegrate and eliminate these toxins, which often enter the general blood circulation. If these toxins enter the brain, they can produce disorientation, confusion or even coma. For this reason, the colon must be cleared of all fecal residue within twenty-four hours after the initial anaphylactic reaction.

The concept that a bowel movement every second or third day is sufficient, is shockingly erroneous. A colon loaded with toxic material damages not only the liver, but the brain as well. Normally the bowels must move once or twice daily. In most instances, the physician will correct this with a proper diet, or recommend a suitable laxative, if necessary.

Dramatic measures are sometimes required to accomplish this, and often an ordinary enema or a high colonic enema may be effective. If either of these treatments do not produce satisfactory results, and an x-ray indicates no obstruction, I use the "old reliable" — 60 cc of castor oil. I have never seen an aggravation of symptoms or other adverse effects with castor oil. On the contrary, I have seen that this dramatic treatment has often changed a depressed, melancholy patient into an optimistic one within hours, eagerly looking forward to his next meal. Such dramatic changes can be experienced when the colonic residue, saturated with bacterial toxins, has been completely eliminated. After the body has been freed of the initial build-up of toxins in the colon, the liver is able to begin its process of self-regeneration. After several days, the patient may begin to eat solid food once more.

Food for Liver Healing

What is the most suitable diet for healing and recovery after the liver suffers an anaphylactic reaction to food? In answering this question, the basic rule to follow is to consume only those foods which cause no allergic or anaphylactic liver reaction of any kind, and which will produce no abdominal discomfort after meals. This is a rule that should be followed throughout life. If there is a marked sense of fullness or pain after eating, the person probably has eaten the wrong kind of food, and such food should be avoided. With the exception of organic disease (which requires the attention of a physician) any abdominal discomfort after meals indicates liver cell sensitivity to that particular food item. Some of the outstanding gastrointestinal manifestations of the anaphylactic reaction of the liver include:

— an uncomfortable abdominal fullness after meals;
— belching of gas;
— abdominal pain, pain between the shoulder blades, backache or neck pain;
— disagreeable taste or breath, canker sores, coated tongue;
— nausea or vomiting; and
— diarrhea or constipation.

The best solid food to be eaten after fasting should be some kind of cooked cereal that is best tolerated by the patient, such as rice, wheat, oatmeal or barley. A little milk and sweetener may be added to the cereal and tea. Coffee and toast with butter can be consumed in moderation. The size of the portions and the frequency of meals can be gradually increased with the patient's tolerance to food. The gastrointestinal tract (including the liver) will heal faster with six smaller helpings than with three larger meals.

This transitional diet should be adhered to for at least three to five days, depending on the speed of recovery. During that time, I recommend that the patient continue to drink from four to six glasses of water daily. If by chance there is an unexplained discomfort after meals, extra glasses of water at room temperature often bring relief.

Why are cooked cereals used to help restore a depressed liver function? In my experience, I have found that the injured liver is able to metabolize cereals before it can metabolize fruits and vegetables. This is also seen in the growing baby when it begins to metabolize solid food. After breast milk, the first solid food tolerated by its developing liver is cooked cereals. Some patients react allergically to some particular vegetable or fruit, which must be eliminated from the diet.

After three to four days, some patients may advance to eating cooked vegetables and fruit, and larger quantities of milk, especially if the anaphylactic reaction of the liver has been a mild one. On the other hand, if the victim has experienced a strong anaphylactic reaction and a variety of food items have been offered too soon, the weakened liver cells may react anaphylactically to one or two of the vegetables or fruits ingested. Such a reaction is always accompanied by liver cell anoxia (insufficient oxygen) which will affect millions of liver cells. In mild disturbances, these cells will then become depressed in function, while in serious cases, many cells may be destroyed and recovery will require patience and time.

This kind of reaction may cause the victim to again

experience abdominal cramps, vomiting and diarrhea, and a week-long effort towards recovery will be ruined. At this point, the patient has to begin the curative process all over again, and drink water with honey from one to two days before solid food is again tolerated. It is important to remember that two or three varieties of simple cereals should be eaten when we want to help the liver to heal itself. After a week we can add different kinds of cooked vegetables and fruit, any cereal, cheese and eggs one by one at first, in small portions, to see whether or not they will cause an allergic reaction. During subsequent weeks, increase both the variety and the quantity of these foods. Eliminate any food item that brings about abdominal pain or discomfort. Although such a "pick and choose" process may pose an inconvenience for a few weeks, the lifelong benefits of freedom from anaphylactic reactions are well worth the trouble.

Prevention: A Primary Approach

In the preceding pages we have discussed the methods of healing an injured liver, and in this section we will study how we can prevent liver injury in the first place. In considering this issue, we need to go back to the first few months of childhood, and examine the first symptoms of food allergy and how they appear.

I have never seen an instance where a newborn baby was allergic to its mother's milk. Apparently at that age, the baby is so much the image of the mother that no antibodies have developed. However, if the mother's milk is not available, the difficulty with an allergic reaction can manifest itself. Some infants are sensitive to cow's milk, and react allergically with abdominal cramps, vomiting, diarrhea or constipation. When this occurs, the doctor will often suggest that the baby be given a commercially prepared vegetable milk, made from soy or other sources, which the infant may tolerate. If the problem is not easily solved, an allergist should be consulted.

Infants and small children often suffer allergic reactions to other foods, and their symptoms usually manifest themselves in functional gastrointestinal, lung and skin disorders. These allergic reactions are more common than bacterial infections and keep both the parents and the pediatrician busy, as they try to identify and eliminate the offending cause.

Infants, while still unable to express their allergic reactions outwardly, will often refuse to eat certain food items such as meat, fruit or vegetables because of the discomfort they cause. Very often a distressed mother will come into the doctor's office, concerned over the youngster's refusal to eat "good food". In most cases, the doctor will side with the child. The mother is often instructed to offer the child nourishing foods, but to respect the child's symptoms of allergic reaction as well. Once the mother becomes aware of the possibilities of anaphylactic food reactions of the liver, her alert and close observation can help avoid such disturbances. She will then reap the reward of an active child who enjoys a happy temperament and exuberant health.

This kind of awareness should continue until adolescence, when the youngster will be able to assume personal responsibility to detect any allergic reactions to food. However, social pressures and the desire for popular foods will often tempt the young boy or girl to eat foods (such as hotdogs and hamburgers) that may cause an anaphylactic reaction of the liver. Although many times no symptoms will appear after such foods are eaten, at other times there will be abdominal cramps, vomiting and diarrhea. A period of weakness, fatique or even anemia may follow such food disturbances. Recuperation may take from one to three days, depending on the severity of the reaction.

Strong anaphylactic reactions of the liver to meat or fats may happen rarely or frequently, depending on the sensitivity of the individual. They are usually dismissed by relatives or doctors as minor food disturbance, ("next time, just watch what you eat") and the incident is promptly forgotten, not realizing that a serious injury to the liver and gastrointestinal tract has just taken place. The victim may sometimes develop secondary signs of deterioration such as weakness, irritability, fatigue, nervousness, depression, headache, defective visions, and the inability to function well in school. Such anaphylactic food reactions of the liver are extremely important to understand. With each repeated attack, there can be progressive microscopic scarring possible, with some irreversible cell destruction.

Eating Meat: Making the Best of It

As stated in the chapter on anaphylaxis, animal proteins from denatured meat cause the strongest allergic reactions of the liver. Even if we assume that the slaughtered animal was in the best of health, and was free of all drugs (such as antibiotics and hormones), the meat is always exposed to air, from the time the animal is slaughtered until it lands on the dinner table to be eaten. As we know, meat is oxidized by air, especially after it has been cooked for the first time. Chemical change takes place in both the fat and lean meat, while denatured by oxidation. *(150-154)* Food scientists have isolated melonaldehyde as one chemical appearing during oxidation; and others are often present as well. *(45-46)* Oxidation increases in quantity with the time the meat is exposed to air. The liver cell reacts to these products of oxidation, anaphylactically. Refrigeration will not completely prevent oxidation, although a low-temperature will tend to slow it down. Once the meat has become denatured by oxidation, no amount of high-temperature cooking will restore it. For this reason, no meat of any kind should be eaten by older people, and those of any age with known coronary disease.

The adolescent boy or girl may not show any allergic reactions when they eat denatured meat. However, if traces of atherosclerosis are found by the time a person is 40 years old, we can assume that the early symptoms of degenerative disease are already beginning to manifest themselves, even though youthfulness will compensate and hide most symptoms for awhile. As the years advance, the degenerative diseases gradually begin to manifest themselves, depending on the individual. One may become afflicted with high blood pressure, the other with gout, another with diabetes, while another may suffer a heart attack or a stroke. Sudden heart attacks or strokes can usually be attributed to an allergic reaction to some food. Meats are the most common causes. One person will begin to weaken gradually with obstructive lung disease, while another will suffer from kidney failure. Often these diseases can be indirectly traced to liver dysfunction that often can be avoided through a prudent vegetarian diet.

However, many people are not willing to adopt such a diet, although some will choose to decrease their intake of meat and increase their consumption of plant foods. For younger people who insist on meat, we will briefly deal with what special care should be used. If heart disease in family, individuals forty years or over should always realize the risk they are taking and should avoid eating any meat in order to avoid a cardiovascular accident with invalidism or death. For those under forty years, the following is advised:

Fish

Freshly caught fish is the easiest meat to digest. It remains fresh for about four hours after it is caught, when it is exposed to normal temperatures. After four hours, a process of spoilage or oxidation begins due to the digestive enzymes found in the muscle tissue. After fish is cooked and exposed to air for any length of time, the oxidation and accumulation of melonaldehyde will cause further denaturization and spoilage. Anaphylactic reactions of the liver due to the chemical changes associated with denaturization are always possible, and should be avoided at all costs. Fish is the most unstable meat, and must be fresh to be safe. Anyone suffering with coronary atherosclerosis should avoid even this lighter meat in their diet.

In order to reduce such spoilage to a minimum for other individuals, the fish should be stored frozen in ice, inaccessible to air, as soon as it is caught, and should be eaten within twenty-four hours. If the fish is canned immediately after it is caught and dressed, it will also be safer to eat, although not as safe as freshly caught fish. Under no circumstances should cooked leftover fish be eaten the next day, as the denaturization process by air is then already far advanced.

Poultry

Ideally, fowl should be brought into the kitchen for cooking just after it is slaughtered. As this is not possible, the bird should be packaged in plastic immediately after dressing, so as to exclude all air, and thus prevent the oxidation and denaturization of the meat. The atherosclerotic consumer must not eat any stored poultry. If packed to exclude air, only those under forty may eat it.

Turkey meat must be mentioned separately because, in my experience, the anaphylactic reactions to denatured turkey meat are more frequent and more severe than with any other fowl. It should never be eaten by the arteriosclerotics over forty years old. The cause may also be the accumulation of melonaldehyde after slaughter. The statistical evidence is overwhelming. The younger consumers should know that the ana phylactic reactions of the liver to any kind of poultry meat are about the same when the fresh meat is cooked and served hot. However, the difference between the anaphylactic reactions due to turkey meat, as compared with other poultry, is greatest when the meat has been stored or refrigerated for even a few days after cooking. I have never seen such violent anaphylactic reactions with chicken, duck or goose as I have with turkey, whether eaten simply with gravy or in a sandwich or casserole. Even the stuffing or gravy without the meat, when heated and consumed the next day or later, can produce severe anaphylactic reactions.

Red Meat

It should never be eaten by anyone with known heart disease, or any person over thirty-eight to forty years of age. For others, I have found no general difference in the anaphylactic reactions of the liver to beef, lamb or pork, although I find them to vary among individuals. Some may develop sensitivities to beef, while others may be allergic to lamb or pork. However, the violence of the reaction of the liver depends on how sensitive the victim's liver cells are to the particular meat, and the size of the portion he or she consumes. In addition, the intensity of the anaphylactic reaction of the liver would also depend on the degree of the degradation and the accumulation of melonaldehyde by the oxidation of the particular meat.

We have no records or observations regarding absolutely fresh meat, because it is not on the market. However, the fresher the meat and the sooner it is served after cooking, the less severe the anaphylactic reaction will be. In theory, if the meat were cooked two or three hours after the animal were slaughtered, and served soon after cooking, the less chance we will have of any anaphylactic liver reaction.

Those who need to be most concerned about anaphylactic reactions are those thirty years of age or older. People who are overweight, who smoke, or who work at a sedentary occupation are often the first to suffer from coronary heart attacks or strokes. They are also the most susceptible to a dangerous anaphylactic liver reaction. Those with a suitable meatless diet, who lose weight, quit smoking, and begin a program of regular physical exercise, are often given a chance to change their bad habits, and reduce the risk of coronary heart attack. However, such a period of grace may not be given to those who consistently sit down to big meals, richly laden with meats and meat fats. With such risks, disaster can strike suddenly and without warning, and a happy dinner party can end abruptly with a heart or stroke tragedy.

For Those Over 40:
Laboratory Tests that are Advisable

One of the most effective methods which can alert a person to a possible risk of heart disease is the High Density Lipoprotein (HDL) cholesterol blood test, which any doctor can arrange. This modern and relatively simple procedure has been found to be more reliable in predicting the true stage of atherosclerotic heart disease or stroke than either the standard blood cholesterol or the tryglyceride tests alone that are so popular today.

Also of practical importance is the Exercise Stress Test, easily arranged by a doctor. The Blood Test and Exercise Stress Test should reveal to the doctor, the correct condition of the patient, and advise him accordingly.

After all the hazardous habits and conditions have been discontinued, both diet and physical exertion have been found of greatest importance to change the HDL level, ideally closer to 70 or higher. And what is the nature of the diet? It is a prudent diet of vegetables, fruit, cereals, legumes, seeds, nuts, low fat dairy products, and the white of egg, provided that the person, by trial, is not sensitive to any of these foods. If so, it could also cause a moderate anaphylactic reaction of the liver, and must be eliminated. Such a diet will help to raise the HDL closer to normal. When making such a statement, we assume that the other conditions of not smoking, weight loss if necessary, regular physical activity, normal blood sugar, and blood pressure, have been maintained. If heart disease in family, those forty years or older should not risk their life by eating meat of any kind.

To those who are aware of the risk involved and insist that they must eat some meat, I would give the following advice: Once you have arrived at a HDL close to 70, try some helpings of very fresh fish, fowl and lean meat twice a week. Then, after four months, have the HDL checked again. By the results, you will know which diet to follow. Your aim must always be to have a HDL close to 70, or higher.

It is likely that with the eating of meat, the HDL will slump down to a lower number again. Such a number puts the patient in the average risk of an ischemic heart attack or stroke. We must also assume that some, by the time they started the prudent diet, have already suffered from advanced atherosclerosis. In order to cause a reversal of the hardening of the arteries and clear them of the fat deposits in the arteries, we must maintain a HDL of 70 or higher. A reversal of atherosclerosis cannot be accomplished with an HDL of 50 to 60, or even less.

I would warn anyone in a serious risk category of an HDL of 35 to 40 or less, to forget about hankering after any meats. It is your life that is at stake. There is abundant documented evidence that the prudent vegetarian diet is sufficient for the maintenance of weight and energy, and at the same time, help to raise the HDL to a favourable level. Such a way of life takes determination and discipline. Observe the confirmed alcoholic and smoker: if firm abstinence is practiced, the craving for alcohol and cigarettes is soon gone. In my experience, this is also true when patients abstain from meat and fats. In a short time, they do not miss these food items, and are happy with their vegetarian-oriented diet.

The Prudent Vegetarian Diet

The vegetarian diet, with some exceptions, is more easily tolerated by the digestive organs than meat and animal fats. If there is any anaphylactic reaction to a vegetarian diet, it is usually mild. Any vegetables, fruits, cereals or nuts that cause such a reaction must also be eliminated. The food eaten must always be agreeable to the digestive organs, and cause no symptoms such as pain, gas, nausea, vomiting, diarrhea or constipation.

Fruit

Fruits, although low in protein, cause very little, if

any, anaphylactic disturbance. There is a difference in tolerance between fresh and cooked fruit. Fresh fruit is always richer in food value, and for this reason is preferred. However, if elderly patients with some digestive dysfunction are disturbed with an anaphylactic reaction with fresh fruit, they often can enjoy the same fruit when it is cooked. Apparently, cooking destroys the allergens, making it less reactive to the liver. For those who can tolerate fresh fruit, it is always preferable. Citrus fruits such as oranges, lemons, grapefruit and pineapple, have been found to cause the least anaphylactic reactions. But all of these food items must be observed one by one, then eliminate the offending item.

Dried Fruit

Dried fruit is a better source of energy, minerals and vitamins than fresh fruit, and should form part of the daily menu. Although fresh fruit may provide more dietary fiber, dried fruit is more effective for its laxative properties.

Vegetables

Leafy vegetables are rich in minerals and vitamins, but low in carbohydrates. They are usually well-tolerated, even by those who have a sensitive digestive system. Root vegetables, besides supplying us with minerals and vitamins, provide us with carbohydrates for energy. The most common on this continent are potatoes, beets, carrots, turnips and radishes.

Pulses are found in two forms: green and dried. They not only have a high carbohydrate content, but protein, vitamins and minerals as well. The most common pulses include beans (pinto, red kidney, soy), peas (both green and yellow), and lentils. For those who follow a prudent diet, legumes (eaten with grains) supply much of their protein requirements.

Nuts

Nuts are rich in both carbohydrates and proteins. They also contain some fat. The anthropoid apes live on fruit and nuts. Evidently they obtain all the protein they require from nuts, since the protein content of fruits are minimal.

Cereals

Cereals are our main source of energy. They are high in carbohydrates, moderate in protein, and provide some fat as well. A patient recovering from a liver injury should adopt a high carbohydrate, low-fat and low-protein diet. Any cooked cereal, fortified with about one pint of milk daily, should provide this perfect combination. Such a diet should be continued for six to fourteen days to give the liver time for healing before other foods are gradually added.

A prudent vegetarian diet is one that provides the protein, fat, carbohydrate, fiber, vitamins and minerals we require daily. Such a diet would basically include a variety of whole grains, legumes, raw nuts and seeds, fruits and vegetables (especially some green leafy ones). Peanut butter and wheat germ make good additions, as does a few tablespoons of brewer's yeast. If one uses dairy products and eggs as well, meeting all nutritional requirements should be a simple task. By monitoring the HDL of the patient, the doctor may have to adjust the diet as to the fat content of the dairy products, and decide whether whole eggs or egg whites alone should be allowed. Whether we choose an all plant (vegan) diet, or a lacto, or lacto-ovo, vegetarian diet (including dairy products and eggs), we will be well on the way towards reaching the desired high HDL.

What to Eat If You Don't Eat Meat
Some High Protein Suggestions:
Beans and Other Legumes
Soybeans, lentils, garbanzos, navy beans, limas, split peas, bean sprouts. They can be used in soups, casseroles, salads, loaves, dips, and sauces.

Grains and Cereals
Wheat and wheat germ, rolled oats, barley, rice, millet, corn. Especially good for pancakes and waffles, grits, mush, oatmeal, wholegrain breads, and dinner loaves. When combined with ordinary or soybean milk, grains and cereal products, provide a very good combination of proteins.

Dairy Products
Eggs, milk, buttermilk, sour cream, cheese (cottage, cream, cheddar), yogurt, ice cream. Recipes using these foods include omelettes (cheese, herb, mushroom, onion, jelly), quiche Lorraine, souffles (cheese, spinach, chocolate), soups (cream of mushroom, potato, asparagus), breads and pastry, Welsh rarebit, macaroni and cheese, cheese or egg salad sandwiches, cheese sauce for vegetables, cheese blintzes, pizza, cheese and eggs in salads or alone. Dairy products also

enhance the nutritional value of casseroles, dinner loaves and sauces.

Nuts and Seeds

Almonds, pecans, walnuts, brazil nuts, filberts, cashews, peanuts, sesame, sunflower and pumpkin seeds; pine nuts (pinon). Can be eaten cooked or raw, and combined with fruits and vegetables in salads, or cooked in loaves, casseroles, breads, soups, and cereals. Nuts and seeds are delicious when eaten raw by themselves.

Your HDL/cholesterol blood test will guide your doctor as to how much fat should be allowed in your diet. He may permit only skimmed milk, skimmed milk cheese, and the white of eggs, if the fat content of your blood is too high.

Additional information about the vegetarian way of life can be found among the periodicals and books dealing with a vegetarian diet. If we were to include such information here, this volume would probably be double its present size. This volume will provide a better understanding of the dangers to some people involved in eating meat and any food they are sensitive to. They will reap the benefits of a prudent vegetarian diet. Humanity will be able to enjoy a healthier and extended life.

CHAPTER SIX

THE LIVER AND EXERCISE

In many parts of the world, the concept of physical exercise is fairly meaningless. In countless villages of India, Latin America, Africa and Asia (as well as the rural areas of many developed countries) millions of men and women regularly perform strenuous physical labor in order to survive. In contrast, many of us live in urban and suburban areas, and are making use of labor-saving devices that were previously not available. Although much of the work of the middle class Americans or Canadians is psychologically exhausting, it requires little or no physical effort. For this reason, these people don't get the necessary exercise at their place of employment.

There is an inescapable law which governs our body that demands that the main portion of the food we eat must be metabolized into muscular work. *(135)* Since mental and emotional stress require only a small part of our food, the main unused portion of a meal becomes a toxic overload to the physically inactive person. Men and women who earn their living by hard muscular work — such as miners, farmers, gardeners and day labourers — easily conform to this law and its requirement. But for office workers, doctors, lawyers and teachers, this is not the case. Therefore, they must devote a certain amount of time each day for strenuous muscular exercise. *(132,134,136)* We have a vague idea that exercise is important. But exactly why is it necessary, and what does it do for us?

The Benefits of Exercise

We all know that bones and muscles form the main part of the human body. The bones, of course, give support to the body and protect many delicate organs (such as the brain, kidneys and liver) from injury. The role of the muscles is twofold. They make our body move, also pump the blood back to the heart, through repeated contractions. At rest, only 5000 to 6000 cc (approximately 5 to 6 quarts) of blood are circulating through the body each minute. During strenuous physical exercise, this circulating volume increases to 24,000 cc (24 quarts) per minute. *(156, pages 221-222)* This dramatic increase in the circulating blood volume is due to the more frequent and stronger contractions of the heart. This flow is also sustained by the strong and frequent contractions of the muscles of the body, which is speedily pumping the blood back to the heart. In other words, the heart pumps oxygen-rich blood throughout the entire body, and the body muscles, by contracting, push the "used" blood back to the heart. Both actions are required for optimum circulation.

There are many benefits to physical activity. The most positive is that the heart and skeletal muscles become stronger with use. With regular exercise, the muscles develop new capillaries and larger arteriolar branches leading to them. These newly developed blood vessels are especially important for the heart because an extra developed supply of blood to the heart muscle benefits the whole body, as well as the heart.

When compared to a state of rest, about four to five times more blood profuses every cell of the body during exercise. This additional circulating blood has a revitalizing effect on every cell in the body. The blood circulation of people who have a sedentary lifestyle is about 5000 cc per minute during the active day; less at rest. *(156, page 221)* As a consequence, a polluted or "rusty" metabolism can result during inactivity. When the metabolic rate is reduced by a long rest, the speedy oxidation and removal of body wastes become stagnant. This causes the metabolic end products to become toxic. Consequently, every cell in the body will eventually suffer. It accounts for the sore and stiff muscles, on rising, in the morning. A depressed metabolism also makes us susceptible to a number of degenerative diseases such as coronary heart disease, diabetes, high blood pressure, stroke and rheumatism. Furthermore, neuropsychiatric complications may follow, such as depression, lack of concentration and loss of memory. Regular exercise and a prudent diet can do much to prevent these problems, and enhance the enjoyment of our lives every single day. *(137-140)*

One important benefit of regular physical exercise is that the blood moves faster. Of equal importance is the larger amount of available blood for the entire muscular system. As the muscles begin to contract with sustained exercise, their blood vessels dilate because of the increased local demand of oxygen and nutrients. This process, in turn, causes the blood to gradually shift from the abdomen (where it normally tends to settle in sedentary individuals) to the activated muscles of the chest, back, arms, and legs. *(157, page 464)* During rest, these muscles receive approximately 2000 cc of the circulating blood per minute. The remaining 3000 cc move slowly through the abdomen. During strong exercise, the supply to the muscles is increased to over 20,000 cc of blood per minute, while the abdomen's supply is reduced to 600 cc. *(157, page 464)* When every cell of the body is profused with larger amounts of oxygen-rich blood, the individual will enjoy greater stamina, greater emotional balance, and increased productivity. It is our natural state to be active. The benefits of regular, dynamic exercise can attest to this, both now and in later years.

Another major benefit of regular exercise is an increase in what is called **stroke volume**. When a trained athlete is at rest, it is not uncommon to find a heartbeat rate of 60 per minute, against the 80 - 100 beats per minute of the untrained, sedentary worker. *(156, pages 221-226)* The stronger heart muscle of the athlete can circulate the blood with a larger filling capacity and stronger (yet slower) contractions; while the sedentary person does so poorly, with faster and weaker contractions. Physiologists state that the stroke volume (the "scoop" of blood with each contraction) of the sedentary person is 50 - 80 cc, whereas the trained athlete enjoys a stroke volume of 200 cc. *(156, pages 221-222)* This means that, with regular strenuous exercises, the stroke volume will increase, assuring even when the body is resting, an optimal circulating blood volume.

When we speak of stroke volume, we also must mention that, in oxygen consumption, there is a great difference between an athlete and a sedentary individual. The physically inactive person uses an estimated 20 cc of oxygen per kilo of body weight per minute. Hence, a sedentary individual weighing 70 kilos (154 pounds) uses approximately 1400 cc of oxygen per minute. On the other hand, a training athlete utilizes 85 cc per kilo of body weight per minute. Taking a person weighing 70 kilos, 5950 cc of oxygen are used. *(156, page 222)* It should be easy to understand that all the metabolic processes of every cell are strongly stimulated by such a large volume of oxygen and nutrients. Nothing but good must follow. This increased metabolic stimulation by regular exercise must revitalize all bodily functions, and help keep it from degenerative disease. We cannot all become athletes, but with increased exercise, we will also be vitalized by an increased oxygen metabolism that will benefit young and old in every walk of life.

People who perform regular muscular work for their livelihood are able to enjoy the lasting benefits that regular exercise provides. However, when they reach retirement age, the pitfall of ill health can suddenly overcome them. Every doctor has witnessed the many tragedies that befall men after they reach retirement age. Women seem more immune to such problems. Even if they retire from gainful employment, they usually remain more active, on their feet at home. Unless a man knows how to retain his physical activity and change to a lighter diet with retirement, he runs a great risk of becoming a victim of a stroke or heart attack. *(141)* Speaking as a medical doctor, it is extremely sad to see men with long and useful lives suddenly die or become disabled invalids, after years of having looked forward to travel, hobbies, being with friends, study ... activities that they were not able to enjoy as much during their working years. Because they do not know how to adjust themselves to a disciplined lifestyle at retirement of a lighter diet and regular exercise, they suddenly become invalids or die with a heart attack or stroke.

Excessive food and lack of exercise are the major causes of such tragedies. *(142-144)* The normal working man was used to eating heavy "he-man" meals, while he engaged in hard muscular work. Upon retirement, he now may lead a sedentary life, and yet continue to eat the same heavy meals. Most likely, these meals would contain generous amounts of meat and animal fats. With such habits, strong anaphylactic reactions of the liver are more likely to occur. Only a well-functioning liver — reaping the benefits of a disciplined diet and exercise, can keep the body clean from accumulating toxins and guarantee a good supply of blood to keep the body functioning at an optimal level.

Some Hidden Problems Connected with Exercise: Second Wind

When inactive, the liver tends to hold a large portion of the circulating blood in the abdomen, *(157, page 464)*, more so during about three to four hours after a meal. When starting to exercise too soon after a meal, the runner seems to labor in breathing for three to five minutes; then experiences a general relief, to proceed with ease. This stage is known as **"second wind"**. It is when the blood shifts from the abdomen into the general musculature, to supply the needed extra volume necessary for running.

The "Pot Belly"

The "**pot belly**", in the male, is the result of the chronically recurring anaphylactic reaction of the liver. Evidence of a habitual abdominal blood congestion is more common with a sedentary lifestyle, rare with the athlete. It can be minimized by habitual exercise and a diet that will not cause an allergic reaction.

Chronic Insomnia

If a person has been physically moderately active before going to bed, he or she will soon sleep. But then in two or three hours, he or she may be wide awake again, no matter how tired. The cause, the reacting swollen liver, (especially after a heavy dinner), prevents a full volume of blood to return to the heart. This also robs the brain of the necessary oxygen and nutrients. Sleep is impossible. The remedy: get up and exercise the arms and legs; (some muscle contractions against a weight) for 3 to 5 minutes. On returning to bed, comfortable sleep will soon come. If necessary, on waking again in 2 or 3 hours, repeat the same exercise, and eat milk and biscuits to raise your blood sugar.

For the same reason, breakfast and lunch should be the heavier meals, and dinner light. A prudent light supper, preferably 5 to 6 hours before bedtime, would assure a better sleep, and greatly reduce the heart attacks and strokes during the night. If hungry, have milk and some baking at bedtime.

Exercise: Which is Right for You?

It is a well-known fact that those who work at sedentary jobs should devote between thirty minutes to one hour a day to regular physical exercise. *(145)* At the present time, there are literally dozens of books that are advocating exercise. *(146)* A wide variety of gyms, health clubs and adult-education classes, devoted to such purposes, can be found in nearly every community.

Exercise, if possible, should be made a pleasure and not a drudgery. The type of exercise one chooses should provide enjoyment, as well as good health. Very often people jump into a specialized exercise program, only to become bored and disillusioned with it after a few weeks. Brisk walking or jogging are among the most popular and beneficial exercises. They relieve tension, and improve breathing and blood circulation. They also give us the chance to enjoy our natural surroundings. Bicycling is a good exercise from both the physical and mental point of view. Cycling improves blood circulation, strengthens the back, leg and shoulder muscles, and improves the functioning of the lungs and heart. Jogging is an excellent all-around conditioner, and improves lung capacity, endurance, muscle tone, and overall strength. It improves the circulation, relieves tension, and increases our flexibility and stamina. Other excellent body conditions include swimming, roller and ice skating, golf, tennis, bowling, shuffleboard, rowing, and stair climbing. All forms of exercise must be increased gradually. *(147)* (If you are over fifty or sixty years of age, the opinion of a doctor should be sought before venturing on any strenuous exercise program). *(148)*

A Note of Caution

Patients suffering with any kind of heart trouble must be especially careful to avoid heavier exertion soon after a meal.

The return flow of blood to the heart is then reduced because a greater volume of blood tends to pool in the abdomen after eating, thus any immediate exertion soon after a meal may embarrass the heart. Therefore, no strenuous exercise should be undertaken after meals. A period of easy movement, such as clearing the table or washing dishes, is preferable. This type of activity keeps a desirable balance between both abdominal and general circulation, and the heart is assured a better return flow during a possible allergic crisis. Any heavier exercise program, on the advice of a doctor, should never follow a meal. Allow three or four hours for the digestive process to subside, and then exercise. It will be easier to increase the general circulating blood volume for the revitalization of the body.

CHAPTER SEVEN

SUDDEN VASCULAR DEATH: THE ROLES OF THE LIVER AND ANAPHYLAXIS IN SUDDEN CEREBRO OR VASCULAR INFARCTION

Introduction

Much has been written about how coronary and cerebrovascular atherosclerosis reduces myocardial or cerebral function, and how it increases the risk of myocardial and cerebral infarction. The cardiologists and pathologists describe arterial disease in detail, but are still seeking the cause of "the sudden event" that leads to an acute myocardial or cerebral infarction. A new concept is presented regarding the cause of these vascular events. The anaphylactic reaction of the liver causes these catastrophic events to occur. Experimental evidence and clinical observations are presented. The liver has a strangulating control of the blood circulation when reacting to improper food. With an anaphylactic reaction of the liver, the return venous flow to the heart is blocked by this organ. At the same time, the coagulative components of the blood are increased, causing myocardial or cerebral infarctions.

1. The Problem

Heart attacks and strokes abruptly terminate almost one million lives each year on the North American continent. The public is helplessly waiting for medical scientists to stem this massive slaughter. This scourge of the twentieth century — this "sudden event" — needlessly blights or ends many active, useful lives below the age of sixty-five. The urgency of the problem is obvious, for myocardial infarction strikes some victim every twenty seconds. It is imperative, therefore, that every possible solution be intensively examined without prejudice *(1-12)* The anaphylactic reaction of the liver is to be blamed as the cause of this great and unnecessary killing. The anaphylactic reaction was clearly documented at the beginning of the twentieth century, yet has been studiously ignored by modern medicine. It should be recognized as the leading reason for most myocardial and cerebral infarctions.

I shall now present the hypothesis in more detail:

The sudden heart deaths that complicate coronary atherosclerosis are caused by an anaphylactic reaction of the liver cells, due to food, or any substance to which the cells are sensitized. By such a reaction, the return flow of blood from the portal vein, the hepatic artery and, in some instances, the inferior vena cava to the heart, is impeded by the swollen, congested liver. With this reaction is associated a drop in blood pressure, a decrease in cardiac output, a hemo-concentration, and an increase of the blood coagulation components. *(4)*

This sudden change in the hemodynamics causes the **ischemia** of the heart muscle and conducting mechanism, especially when the blood in its viscid condition at lowered pressure, meets a stenotic coronary artery. *(5,105-109)* All varieties of cardiac arrhythmias, including fibrillation, all varieties of vascular myocardial damage from focal or diffuse subendocardial coagulative myocytolysis, to transmural coagulative necrosis are simply due to ischemia, dependent in part or altogether, on the intensity and length of the anaphylactic reaction of the liver.

2. The Liver

To the casual observer, the liver is one of the least impressive organs of the body. Dull in color, and with no apparent motion, it weighs 1500 grams, and is comprised of about 1,000,000 lobules, each of which holds 350,000 cells. *(13)* The blood perfuses these cells as it flows through the sinusoids. Because of its enormous metabolic activity, the liver requires 1500 cc of oxygenated blood per minute. This is 25 percent of the body's total blood circulation, and it carries about 20 percent of the total oxygen required by the body. *(14)*

Two main vessels supply the liver with nutrients; the portal vein and the hepatic artery. The blood from these two vessels join before flowing through the millions of microscopic canals called sinusoids. The sinusoidal canals are lined on either side with liver cells, where the blood comes into immediate contact with the cells. The exchange of **metabolites**, the nutrients from the digestive system, also takes place here. In addition, the sinusoids are provided with inlet and outlet **sphincters**, under both **sympathetic** and **vagal** nerve control, which regulate the flow of blood through the liver. *(14a-18)*

The response of the sinusoids to **ephedrine** is dose

dependent, causing constriction of sphincters within ten to thirty minutes. *(15-18)* The function of the sinusoidal canals have been well-documented. They close when the sensitized liver cells, which line the sinusoids, react by swelling to any foreign substance or food in the blood as it flows through the canals. The sinusoidal canals are also closed when the **sphincters**, located on each end of the canals, contract in response to sympathetic nerve stimulation. *(19-22)*

3. **The Anaphylactic Reaction**

The word **anaphylaxis** (ana- against, phylaxis protection) is defined in Dorland's Illustrated Medical Dictionary, as "an unusual or exaggerated allergic reaction of an organism to foreign proteins or other substances." Anaphylaxis is an **antigen-antibody** reaction. The term was originally used to describe an allergic reaction of liver cells in laboratory animals which had been sensitized by injecting a foreign substance such as horse serum. The terms **hypersensitivity reaction, immune reaction** and **foreign protein reaction,** are also used to describe anaphlaxis. This knowledge has been extended to human reactions as well. *(3-5)* Any injection or ingestion of a foreign substance can render some individuals hypersensitive to that same substance at a later time.

The electron-microscope, during the last few decades, permitted direct visual observation of this impressive phenomenon, so that this branch of human physiology could be well-documented. *(23-65)* A typical experiment was described as follows: "A dog was given an injection of 5 cc of horse serum. Two weeks later, he received 20 cc of horse serum intravenously. After the injection, the dog went immediately into acute anaphylactic shock. The dog died within 30 - 60 minutes after the injection of 20 cc of horse serum, in an anaphylactic shock.'' In the post-mortem report, the liver was found to be the main target of the anaphylactic reaction, and was described as follows: "The condition of the liver dominates the pathological impression and presents a picture such as is rarely, if ever, seen under any circumstances. The organ is tremendously swollen. The color is intensely cyanotic, on section, the cut surface bleeds freely. The **Portal Vein** and the **Inferior Cava** are found enlarged with blood.''

The description of the rest of the digestive organs continues: "The gastrointestinal tract is found to be the seat of severe congestion. There is bleeding into the wall of the stomach and intestine, with haemorrhagic diarrhea. The pancreas may show some increased swelling. The spleen is markedly enlarged.'' *(19)* We note, not only is there an acute **Portal hypertension**, but the **Inferior Cava** is obstructed as well. Since the **caudate lobe** is firmly attached to the Cava (anatomists add that in certain cases, the liver substance completely encircles the **Vena Cava**), enlargement of this organ could also strangle this large blood vessel. *(19)*

Allergists state that during an anaphylactic reaction, sixty percent of the total circulating blood volume can be held in the large and small veins of the abdomen and the lower extremities. When such a reaction occurred in laboratory experiments on dogs, the blood pressure dropped from 138 mm Hg to 44 mm Hg. The cardiac output decreased from a mean of 3.08 L/min.

to .52 L/min. Hemoconcentration occurred with a fifteen percent increase in **hematocrit** reading. *(4)*

4. **Anaphylaxis the Same in Man**

The pathology of the anaphylactic shock in the dog has been documented so thoroughly and frequently, as to become a classic. However, experimental anaphylactic shock in human beings has not been undertaken under laboratory conditions, and the reason is obvious: No one would submit to such experimentation! However, the clinical picture and the **morphological** findings of the anaphylactic shock victims, in all species, including man, are the same. The liver is the main target of the anaphylactic reaction, leading to shock. For instance, an irreversible **haemorrhagic shock** cannot be produced experimentally if the liver is excluded from the general circulation. *(52)* Furthermore, the irreversibility of the haemorrhagic shock can be prevented by **viviperfusion** of the liver, while the rest of the body is held in a **hypotensive** and **hypovolemic** state for up to seven and one-half hours. The damage to the central nervous system during this time is minimal and transitory. *(57)* Experimentally then, it has been proven without a doubt, that the liver is the dominating organ in irreversible shock.

During the first half of this century, **clinicians** were satisfied that this reaction was similar in both animals and humans. There are several reports that support such a concept. For instance, when a pathologist performs a post-mortem examination of the liver involved in an anaphylactic reaction, he will, at times, find the engorged organ swollen with blood and edema. In other instances, the edema may have dissipated, and all he finds is **central necrosis**. *(56)* How is this related to the anaphylactic reaction? During the height of the anaphylactic reaction, the sinusoids are closed, with the liver cells swollen. At the periphery of the lobule, where the blood enters, the cells may still be well-oxygenated. However, the central portion of the lobule receives **anoxic blood**, due to the swollen liver cells which close the sinusoids. Therefore, these central cells die first, and those at the periphery, die last. For this reason, with an anaphylactic reaction, central necrosis is a common post-mortem finding in animals, as well as in man. Many pathologists do not find this because they do not look for it.

Some patients with severe superficial burns will die from irreversible anaphylactic shock as soon as local treatment, such as moving the **eschar**, is started. *(58,64)* Such a reaction could have the following explanation: Upon admission to the hospital, as long as the injured tissue is fixed locally, very little **necrotic** material enters the circulation, and the patient remains stable. But when an attempt is made to remove the eschar, the **denatured** protein molecules (i.e. products of the burn) enter the circulatory system. They are carried to the liver, and as they pass through the sinusoids, cause the anaphylaxis. The authors that report these findings conclude that anaphylactic liver reactions to denatured proteins are the same in humans, as when produced in the dog experimentally. *(58,64)*

Traumatic or crushed muscle shock is similar in its

pathophysiology. As such, it has been documented experimentally in animals, and clinically in humans. *(57)* When a large enough portion of muscle tissue has been crushed, irreversible shock may follow. The mascerated muscle tissue becomes necrotic due to local anoxia, and acts as foreign protein. When these foreign protein molecules enter the sinusoids, the liver cells react with **edematous** swelling, thereby closing the sinusoidal blood channels. Crushed muscle tissue cause the same type of shock both in animals and human beings due to anaphylaxis.

Similar examples include a soldier who received prophylactic injections of anti-tetanus serum (he died in an anaphylactic shock within one hour); (See also *(61)* insect *(62)* stings, estrogen *(66)* injections, and oral *(67)* penicillin administration.) *(63,69,70)* Since the liver is the **detoxifying** organ of the body, all foreign substances arrive there first to be assimilated or broken-up and expelled from the body. There is little difference whether the foreign substance or antigen enters orally or **parenterally**. The reaction is the same, except that when the parenteral injection is administered, the body reacts more speedily. The autopsy of these victims revealed the same gross and microscopic changes in the liver that were found in experimental animals after a fatal anaphylactic reaction of the liver.

Although there is strong evidence that clinically, there is no difference between animal and humans with regard to the anaphylactic reaction, we shall briefly note the various other theories that have been proposed regarding the mechanism and cause of the anaphylactic shock in humans with no supportive proof.

5. Various Theories Regarding the Cause of Anaphylactic Reaction

All theorists agree that the alarming decrease in blood volume in connection with shock causes an irreversible deterioration of all body functions and subsequent death. **"Hypotension"** as the cause, is expected with the decrease in blood volume. **"Hemoconcentration"** as the cause, is due to excessive loss of plasma, part of the anaphylactic reaction (the thoracic duct carries eight times the normal lymph during the early phase of shock). It will cause a decrease in blood volume and hemoconcentration. *(53,54)* **"Laryngeal edema"** as the cause, can be overcome by tracheotomy, and cannot cause an irreversible loss of blood volume found in shock.

"Bronchial spasm" is also mentioned as a cause. How could one explain the loss of blood volume by bronchial spasm? It can be a secondary effect. Some mention **"Splanchnic pooling"** as the cause of an anaphylactic shock. But what is the cause of the splanchnic pooling? It is a consequence of the anaphylactic reaction of the liver and not the cause. It is the result of the closure of the sinusoids of the liver during the anaphylactic reaction. The mesenteric and hepatic arteries pump the blood into the "splanchnic pool", while the venous (Portal) return flow of blood to the heart is impeded by millions of reacting sinusoids. The "splanchnic pooling" concept supports the hypothesis that the liver is the target organ in anaphylactic shock. However, hypotension, hemocentration, laryngeal edema and bronchial spasm are the expected effects, and not the cause of the anaphylactic reaction of the liver.

6. The Anaphylactic Reaction Can Damage the Heart

In experiments on dogs, "Myocardial Failure" is frequently mentioned as a major factor in the irreversibility of the anaphylactic shock. *(5-7)* This can be expected, when in an anaphylactic shock, we observe a critical insufficient coronary profusion due to marked hemoconcentration, accompanied by a drop in blood pressure from a mean of 138 mm Hg to 44 mm HG, with a decreased cardiac output from a mean of 3.08 L/min. to .52 L/min. *(4)* Pathologists describe the myocardium of these experimental animals with such terms as: "myofibrils are swollen", "transverse bands decreased", "contraction of myocytes at the intercalated disks", "sacromeres are disrupted", "myofilaments are distorted and displaced" and "mitrochondria are absent." *(2-4)* These descriptions are evidence of hypoxic **myocardial deterioration**, due to hypotension and hypovolemia. *(95-98)*

7. Denatured Food Causes the Anaphylactic Reaction in Man

Food is the main cause of an anaphylactic reaction in humans, and is of primary interest in this discussion. The reaction to food varies in intensity. Denatured meat (including red meats, poultry, and fish) can provoke the strongest immune reactions. Food scientists have shown that oxidation changes meat to a denatured condition. Melonaldehyde has been found to be one end product of meat oxidation. The reaction of the liver cells may be due to this chemical. *(45-46)* The liver cells in some patients may become sensitized to these oxidative products of meat, and react when meat is ingested. Any food or foreign substance may cause such an anaphylactic or immune reaction, but not nearly as frequently or severely as meat or meat products.

8. Anaphylactic Reaction May Vary in Strength

It is the prevailing opinion that an anaphylactic reaction is always violent, and can even be fatal. In fact, allergic, immune, anaphylactic, or foreign protein reactions, can vary considerably. Some can be fatal, others mild, depending on the antibody build-up, and how much antigen has entered the body by injection or ingestion. Such reactions are often associated with a disturbed blood circulation. A strong reaction may lead to irreversible shock, whereas, a minor circulatory disturbance due to anaphylaxis, may pass with a fleeting spell of "light-headedness" due to the associated hypotension. Allergists also agree that when an acute anaphylactic shock occurs, up to sixty-six percent of the blood volume can be kept out of circulation by the liver. *(55)*

9. Myocardial Damage Without Coronary Thrombosis

During an anaphylactic reaction, it is easy to imagine how the blood perfusion of the myocardium by the coronary arteries must be critically reduced. *(99-104)* This **histo-pathological** description of such **myofibers**, when they deteriorate with anoxia, have been well-documented experimentally, and confirmed as postmortem findings in sudden deaths. *(4a, 105-109)* The coagulative myocytolysis can be focal or diffuse, de-

115

pending on the irregularity of the atherosclerotic involvement, and the developed collateral circulation. As expected, the **subendocardium** suffers the first and earliest damage because of the greatest distance from the **epicardium**, which contains the larger coronary arteries. *(110-114)* Furthermore, this hypothesis supports the concept held by some noted cardiologists that the myocardial infarction precedes the **occlusive coronary thrombosis** in many instances. *(4a,115-118)* In other words, the occlusive coronary thrombosis is a secondary, rather than a causative or primary event. *(119-121)*

10. Myocardial Ischemia Causes Sudden Heart Deaths

Outstanding cardiologists of this century continue to debate the cause of the sudden heart deaths. *(79-86)* There are those who hold that a thrombotic occlusion, of one or more coronary arteries, causes the myocardial infarction with or without cardiac arrest. *(94)* This concept does not explain why two-thirds of the sudden heart deaths have no coronary thrombosis. *(4a)* Other researchers have convincing evidence that the first event of a sudden heart death is a **myocardial necrosis**, with or without a secondary coronary thrombosis. Such necrosis is the result of a local ischemia due to a **"circulatory collapse"** of the coronary system without occlusion. These are the findings in two-thirds of the sudden heart deaths reported. *(82,93,100)* An occlusive thrombosis of the coronary arteries was found only in one-third of the sudden heart deaths. With such convincing statistics, the question arises, what causes this sudden ischemia of the heart muscle? Or what produces this sudden "circulatory collapse," *(85,109)* while the coronary arteries are not obstructed? The concept presented in this paper is the answer. With the immune reaction of the liver, the return flow of blood from the lower half of the body (including caval and portal veins) to the heart can be critically reduced. This results in an **acute hypotension** and **hypovolemia** of the coronary system. The effect would be an **ischemic necrosis** of the myocardium, which could end fatally. *(87-92)* This would explain the cause of the sudden cardiac arrest without thrombosis in two-thirds of the reported cases. *(4a)* A short but strong allergic reaction of the liver could have such an effect. A sudden heart death could follow. If the immune reaction of the liver is weaker and more prolonged, the heart muscle contractions could first become weaker and irregular due to ischemia. The resulting stagnant circulation of the myocardium could then progress secondarily causing an occlusive coronary thrombosis; and so, finally end in a **massive transmural infarction** with cardiac arrest. In other words, a sudden heart death can occur with atherosclerotic or normal coronary arteries. Furthermore, it can occur with or without occlusive thrombosis of the coronary arteries, because the final determining factor, in both events, is outside the heart, namely, the length and intensity of the immune reaction of the liver.

11. **Heart Attacks while Victim is Resting**
It is also easier to understand why most sudden heart deaths do not occur after an acute exertion, but at rest,

while the victim is sitting in a chair, or resting on a couch or in bed. *(49)* When a person is inactive or has a sedentary occupation, the blood (especially after a heavy meal, to which he is sensitive) shifts more from the extremities into the **splanchnic pool**. When an anaphylactic reaction of the liver takes place, this pool of blood is trapped in the abdomen. This, in turn, reduces the venous blood flow to the heart more suddenly than if the victim were active and on his feet. If the anaphylactic reaction occurs while he is moderately active, the extremities require a greater portion of the five thousand cubic centimeters of blood per minute that is available to the heart in an adult. Hence, during an anaphylactic reaction, the liver can only trap a smaller volume in the splanchnic pool, while the blood from the extremities and trunk is available and free to return to the heart, unhindered, and thus, sustain the coronary perfusion during the critical moments of the reaction. If the coronary vessels are free of atherosclerosis, it would take an unusually strong reaction to cause an acute ischemic **coagulative myocytolysis** or an ischemia of the **conducting mechanism**, to result in a cardiac arrest. With advanced coronary atherosclerosis, an immune liver reaction need only to be moderate in strength to cause a transmural myocardial infarction with fatal results.

12. Recovery Room Deaths (Anaesthetic)

An example of cardiac arrest with perfectly normal coronary vessels would be the anaesthetic or recovery room heart death, during which, at times, even adolescent patients may succumb. In such instances, the victim's liver might have been sensitive to the anaesthetic or any other drug used in that immediate pre or postoperative period, to which the liver reacts anaphylactically. With such a reaction, the sinusoids of the liver close and block the return flow of blood from the splanchnic pool. Finally, the increased weight of the liver, while resting on the back during the reaction, could further compress the Cava against the firm, muscular, and bony posterior wall. The reduced volume of blood which reaches the heart can be insufficient to sustain the perfusion and viability of the conducting mechanism, and cardiac arrest follows. The anaesthetic department can prevent such deaths by carefully monitoring the patient's sensitivity to drugs and anaesthetics before the operation. Futhermore, always rest the unconscious patient on his or her right side, to lessen the weight of the liver on the caval vein.

Another victim may become sensitized to a drug or anaesthetic at a previous operation. Following this exposure, the antigen (or drug) can produce widespread antibodies throughout the body. When this patient has his second operation, at some later period, using the same drug or anaesthetic, he can have a violent antigen-antibody reaction. If untreated, this can end in a fatal shock.

The "delayed reaction" may occur within 24 to 36 hours after the exposure to that particular anaesthetic. The liver is the main target of this anaphylactic reaction. Experimentally, if the liver is excluded from the antigen, there may be a moderate reaction, which allows much time for treatment to save the life of the victim.

The anaphylaxis takes the following course: Toxic substances with **histamine** are released into the vascular system. The capillaries dilate and allow leakage of plasma into the tissues of the body; the blood pressure consequently drops. The liver is most critically involved in this anaphylactic reaction. Since it is the detoxifying organ of the body, any toxic substance in large concentration generated in the body will arrive at the liver early. The massive quantity of toxic substances overcome the valiant liver cells. With this reaction, the liver cells swell up with edema and close the sinusoid canals. The liver now blocks the return flow of blood from the abdominal viscera to the heart. Normally this amounts to 1500 cc per minute. It is easy to see why the victim deteriorates so rapidly.

The heart fibrillates because of hypoxia due to ischemia of the conducting system. It is impossible to maintain a viable blood pressure at this stage. The patient sinks into coma and death.

In order to prevent such tragedies, the patient considered for a major surgical operation should be "skin tested" for the anaesthetic or drugs to be used. The sensitivity to the anaesthetic could be discovered and that particular anaesthetic avoided. For the post-operative period, the care is usually routine, familiar to the attending staff.

I would like to emphasize a few signs that would warn the attending nurses or doctors of an impending danger. An increased rate of respiration may be due to three causes:

    (a)   Myocardial failure — this can be easily detect ed; or

(b) Anaphylaxis with onset of pulmonary edema — this should be detectable;

(c) Increased respiratory rate due to **hypoxic hepatosis**. The diaphragm rests on the liver. If the liver cells deteriorate due to anoxia, they are very toxic to the surrounding tissues.

With regard to the diaphragm, it will be paralyzed because of the toxicity of the ischemic necrosis of the liver on which the diaphragm rests. Such a patient will be short of breath since only the intercostal muscles are available to relieve his or her air hunger. The diaphragm does not move with respiration because of toxicity.

The attending medical staff will observe these early signs of alarm and begin early treatment for shock. I would warn the staff of the danger of overhydration with intravenous saline administration. Change to Glucose in distilled water immediately. Hypertonic Glucose (10% + 20%), even a vial of 50% can be given. The capillaries by this time have allowed some plasma to exude into the tissues. By using hypertonic glucose solution intravenously, some of this edema can be drawn into the vascular system by osmosis.

General edema disorganizes the normal physiological and chemical process in the body everywhere. For this reason, dehydration carefully monitored is an important measure to overcome the crisis.

13. **Sudden Death Associated with Heavy Exertion**

The history of some patients indicates that the acute myocardial infarction was precipitated by unusual physical exertion. The cause of an infarction is always myocardial ischemia. The ischemia may be due to an occlusive coronary thrombosis or hypovolemia and associated acute hypotension which could be caused by an anaphylactic reaction. When an anaphylactic reaction of the liver to a meal occurs, central cell damage of the liver lobule, with partial closure of the sinusoids with swollen liver cells due to hypoxia, should be looked for. During the time of healing of the lobule (which may take days or weeks) there will be a variable impediment to the venous return flow of blood through the liver. A moderate splanchnic pool can remain, which may last for days. This reduces the total circulating blood volume available. If such a person suddenly exerts himself physically, the muscles of the rest of the body demand extra blood. As the capillaries dilate to supply this blood to the extremities with much of the blood still in the **portal system**, the total return volume can be critically reduced to the embarrassment of the myocardium. When advanced coronary atherosclerotic narrowing is present, an acute cardiac **micro-circulatory** collapse with infarction can occur.

14.   **Cardiac Arrhythmias (Irregularities)**

It is usually accepted that cardiac arrhythmias appear when the **A.V. or S.A. nodes**, or the **conducting mechanism** have suffered ischemic damage. *(4a)* The **extra systoles** may appear gradually, as we would expect with gradually increasing coronary atherosclerosis. It is also observed that a patient, after a heavy dinner, goes to bed with a normal cardiac rhythm, and awakens in the morning with acute cardiac arrhythmia. Such heart injury may follow an anaphylactic reaction of the liver to the meal of the night before. The reaction reduces the venous return to the heart, causing ischemic damage to the nodes and conducting mechanism by a possible focal coagulative **myelocytolysis**. Such conducting injury may be temporary or permanent. It requires the immediate attention of a physician.

15. Anaphylactic Reaction Can Cause Hypercoagulation with Cerebral or Coronary Thombosis

It has been well-documented that, during the first minutes of an anaphylactic reaction, the blood hypercoagulates. However, soon after the initial phase, it is difficult to produce a clot, and the coagulation time is prolonged. At first, there is an increased flow of lymph from the liver into the thoracic duct (measured at 5.45 times the normal flow), which is thought to be due to an increased permeability of the **sinusoidal endothelium**. *(53,54)* This, in part, could account for the increased concentration of red blood cells. The hematocrit reading is elevated. The blood in such viscid state is difficult to move, especially through an **atheromatously** narrowed artery, and could cause a myocardial or cerebral infarction with or without occlusion. An arterial occlusion is, however, possible, since all the various **coagulation** factors such as fibrin, platelets, and thrombin are all increased during the early phase of a strong anaphylactic reaction. *(122-126)*

The anaphylactic reaction, which aroused the interest of scientists during the early part of this century, has almost been forgotten. It is now associated with the rare catastrophic shock reaction due to hemorrhage, a drug or an insect bite. It is not generally realized that, if there is a strong, sometimes fatal, anaphylactic reaction, there must also be countless degrees of less severe minor reactions, since all other allergic reactions vary in intensity. Hence, the only symptom of a minimal anaphylactic reaction of the liver with **portal hypertension**, may be functional dyspepsia. An anaphylaxis of the liver is a problem which everyone experiences at sometime, with heartburn, flatulence, and abdominal cramps; all due to a temporary anaphylactic portal stasis, with hypoxia of the gastrointestinal tract, and associated dysfunction. *(78)*

16. In Order to Appreciate the Enormity of the Anaphylactic Reaction: A Few Suggestions Why the Moderate Anaphylactic Reaction Eludes Notice of the Pathologist

First of all, we must consider the large surface area involved in this reaction. The liver is a unit of thirty-five billion highly specialized cells, nourishing the body, as well as separating and expelling any harmful toxic substances. These cells are grouped into 100,000 lobules each of which have 350,000 liver cells. *(13)* The cells, which are arranged in circling fashion and so form the millions of sinusoidal canals. Each cell faces the blood stream, bare and direct. Although 1500 cc of blood flow through the liver every minute, it is moving at a very low pressure. The portal vein pressure is 8 mm Hg., the **intrahepatic pressure** 4 mm Hg. and the **hepatic vein** blood pressure, 1 mm Hg.

The dynamics of this large surface area with a low pressure propulsion of the blood through the millions of narrow channels are enormous. The whole event in man is a microscopic event, and still has this disastrous effect on heart and brain. The scientist will observe closer and confirm this concept.

The sinusoidal canals are a little wider than a red blood cell. The thirty-five billion liver cells form the walls of these canals. The liver cells, when reacting anaphylactically, need only to expand this microscopic distance to close the canals and make the liver a solid impervious organ. The post-mortem examination, hours or days after death, may reveal no gross striking change of the liver. The evidence is in the microscopic study of the victim's liver.

Secondly, Professor Aschoff, in his text of pathology, differentiates between two causes of central necrosis — a frequent finding in a post-mortem examination, quote:

"In right heart failure with passive congestion of the liver, 'central necrosis' is associated with congestive dilatation of the hepatic vein and its radicals. Whereas in an anaphylactic reaction 'central necrosis' is associated with relatively empty hepatic vein and its tributaries."

To observe these and other important evidences of the anaphylactic reaction of the liver as the cause of the myocardial or cerebral infarctions will require more careful and earlier extra microscopic studies of the victim in the post-mortem room.

CHAPTER EIGHT

LIVER AND ALCOHOL

Every commonly informed adult is aware of the fact that alcoholic beverages can injure the liver. I shall briefly summarize the documentations recorded in the medical textbooks and research literature, together with my own clinical experience with patients who suffered from alcohol abuse.

Physical dependence has been used as a measure for defining alcoholism, also anyone showing withdrawal symptoms if he stops suddenly after a drinking bout of one to two weeks, (such as irritability, tremor, insomnia, anxiety, et cetera). Above all, true alcoholism can be diagnosed when it causes a life problem such as losing a job or threatened divorce proceedings. Furthermore, the victim should have been aware of many warnings that he is ruining his liver and life long before he becomes a true alcoholic, such as periods of depression, associated with a gradual increase in indigestion.

The abuse of alcoholic beverages is especially increasing with young adults. The peak age for alcohol intake causing some problem is between 18 and 25 years. Between 70% - 80% of adults in the United States and Canada drink more than occasionally. The highest percentage of drinkers are the college educated, and affluent Caucasians and Jews. It has become a life problem to 5% - 10% of adult males. The most seriously ill, the "skid row" alcoholic, represents less than 5% of the alcoholic population. The question arises, why do the victims abuse the use of alcohol? We must realize that alcoholism is a disease. No single cause is agreed on. There are social factors, for instance, living with a drinking society. Other causes are a feeling of insufficiency or psychological stress, as depression, in which relief is sought with alcoholic beverages to stimulate or benumb the mind.

Alcohol is a drug which can destroy, or at least temporarily damage, the liver cells. The severity of the damage or actual destruction of the cells depends on the alcohol content of the beverage, the volume drunk, in what period of time. The alcohol abuser often does not remember how much he has been drinking. Furthermore, while drinking, the judgement is poor and it does not take long before much damage to the liver has been done.

Careful medical studies have revealed that even with moderate drinking of alcoholic beverages, the liver cells are damaged. As we know, the liver is the detoxifying organ of the body. It meets this drug as the main target when alcohol is consumed. Investigators have found whenever liver cells are damaged, the finer structures of the cells become paralyzed. As evidence, we notice an accumulation of fat in the cells. Normally the liver cell easily metabolizes the fat, but when the cell is injured by a toxic drug, (in this instance, alcohol) this mechanism of the cell is paralyzed, and fat gradually replaces the whole liver cell. If the alcohol consumption has been moderate, and there are long intervals of abstinence, the liver cells may regenerate to more normal function between the drinking bouts. Hence, the cell injury or destruction depends on the dose and duration of the alcohol intake and the interval time to heal the damage done. With strong abuses, or if the victim unknowingly is highly sensitive (allergic) to even moderate doses of alcoholic beverages, millions of liver cells are being filled with fat. When seen, during an incidental abdominal operation, such liver has a light yellow color. Naturally those liver cells that have been replaced by fat are functionless. That highly complex mechanism with which the liver cell metabolizes and stores our nutrients is arrested and useless.

Since life and exuberant health is moment by moment dependent on good liver function, the whole body will manifest signs of deterioration, even with a moderate degree of liver damage. Of course, with a persistent alcoholic, the damage to the liver cells does not stop by changing them to a fat globule. The damage can progress to an inflammation of the liver (hepatitis), then leading to necrosis (destruction), and irreversible scar formation (cirrhosis). Such change may take from 10 to 15 years.

Even with a moderate liver injury we find frequent long lasting bronchial infections of the lung, which are difficult to treat. Skin rashes and boils will distress the victim frequently. This is the effect of a weakened liver that is unable to detoxify the body and resist infections. Others will suffer with malnutrition, underweight, anemia, lack of vitamins and minerals because the damaged liver cannot assimilate and store these important nutrients in order to maintain robust health. Observe all the degenerative diseases; they increase to the direct extent as the liver deteriorates and fails in function. (Such as high blood presure, atherosclerosis, heart disease, strokes, diabetes, gout, other forms of arthritis, and kidney diseases.) In fact, there is not a cell in the body that is not affected by such depressed liver function. The highly sensitive brain suffers early when perfused with this toxic drug. We all know how easily an alcohol abuser can end up seriously injured or killed in a motor vehicle accident because of his poor judgement and euphoria. Acute intoxication is furthermore associated with tremor, irritability, insomnia, anxiety, agitation, disorientation and even hallucinations, seizures, impotence and acute psychosis. Different nerves and muscles are variably affected, (for instance, weakness in the legs, unsteady gait), so that he soon has to use a cane to prevent himself from stumbling.

The alcohol abuser becomes extremely sensitive to any medication. A doctor has to be very careful in prescribing any medications because the damaged liver metabolizes the medication at different rates in each alcoholic. What is normal dose to the average person may be an overdose to the alcohol abuser.

The miseries of the alcohol abuser are endless. First of all, he must notice how the various faculties of body and mind gradually deteriorate. The gainful work soon suffers. He arrives late for work, or even misses several days following a drinking bout. He was considered an excellent worker, always punctual and dependable, but not now. He is less efficient. He finally loses his job.

His wife loses confidence in his ability to provide for the family. He drinks heavier to overcome the periods of depression. The wife makes every effort, with love and persuasion, to free him from the strangling hold this drug (alcohol) has on him, but to no avail. Finally his behaviour becomes so difficult that the wife fears for her life and that of her children, and leaves the home with the family. If such a man sobers up and contemplates on his ruined life, how he lost his health, his wife and family, his job and reputation, he soon would realize that the more relief he sought in alcoholism, the deeper he sank into difficulties.

However, there is good news for those who wish to turn from such a life of self-destruction to normality again. There are many agencies now assisting those who need help and wish to be rehabilitated again such as Alcoholics Anonymous, group therapy, counsellor consultants, and the prayers of clergymen. In any case, the victim should be assured that delivery from alcoholism is possible.

With regard to the damaged liver cells, this organ is endowed with a remarkable power of regeneration. That is, even though in many areas of the liver only framework of the sinusoids are left, the liver cells will regenerate again. This healing of the liver may take months of patient perseverance, but with the diet given in the chapter of "Healing of the Liver", many of the functions of the liver can be restored again. The mega-vitamins and moderate doses of dehydrocholic acid (bile salts) are a great help in accomplishing this.

CHAPTER NINE

Introduction

Hypoxia of the kidney cells causes general hypertension. Dr. H. Goldblatt discovered that a restricted blood flow, due to a renal artery anomally, causes general high blood pressure. This finding has been accepted by the medical scientists throughout the world.

In this article I call attention to an altogether different renal **hypoxemia**. There is strong clinical evidence that it causes high blood pressure in the majority of hypertensives.

THE CAUSE OF HIGH BLOOD PRESSURE — A NEW HYPOTHESIS

High blood pressure can be reduced, often to normal, by a prudent diet. These experiences are commonly mentioned over the "hot line", and available also in literature. It may take several months of self-discipline to attain the optimum results. The medication that is being used by the patient for hypertension can then usually be gradually eliminated. Every such attempt should be made under close supervision of a medical doctor. That diet alone can control the blood pressure, is well known on this continent. Also, in Asia with a lighter diet, hypertension is very rare. If, however, these Asiatics immigrate to this continent and adopt the American diet, many soon suffer with hypertension, with other American citizens.

The question arises, how does this happen? What explanation can be given? To make this treatment more acceptable to doctors and patients, the probable physiological mechanism involved will be presented.

We are now nearing the end of the twentieth century. Still, the cause of high blood pressure has not been explained. Since it is such a massive killer, most universities throughout the world have concentrated their research studies on the cause of hypertension, especially so during the last century. Every possible explanation, except the one presented in this article, has been studied, yet no physio-chemical cause has been found.

It is the lifestyle of civilization that causes this malady. It prevails mainly in Europe and America. In the third world it is found only where the American or European diet is used. We die prematurely because of the food we eat. By now this observation should be common knowledge. Why has the medical world not accepted it? Because medical scientists have been trained to acknowledge and accept only facts that have been proven to rest on sound physiological principles. These will be presented.

In 1933 Dr. H. Goldblatt published an article in the Journal of Experimental Medicine dealing with the cause of hypertension. His findings were confirmed by medical scientists throughout the world. He found that young individuals, who were born with an obstructive "kink" of the renal (kidney) arteries, developed general hypertension. Such elevated blood pressure would return to normal after this "kink" of the renal artery was released by a surgical operation. What happened: the "kinked" renal artery obstructs the flow of fresh blood required by the kidney cells. As a result, the kidney cells suffered from lack of oxygen. The hypoxic kidney cells then released chemicals into the general circulation, such as renin, angiotensin and aldosterone. These chemicals cause a general **vasoconstriction** resulting in hypertension. Furthermore, the ordinary table salt is then retained in the body, which further increases the blood volume and blood pressure.

The very important discovery of Dr. Goldblatt then is: When kidney cells do not get enough oxygen for their metabolic needs, they release chemicals which cause general hypertension. This very important law of physiology has been accepted and used by the medical world since the year 1933.

After many centuries of diligent research, this is the only cause of hypertension found. After reviewing the accepted physiological principle that renal ischemia causes hypertension, I am presenting another cause of renal ischemia, which can also cause hypertension. And it is likely the main cause of high blood pressure.

Simply then, kidneys suffering damage by lack of oxygen cause high blood pressure. As long as the kidneys get a normal supply of oxygen, the blood pressure remains normal. To this there are rare exceptions: they are certain brain or adrenal gland tumors. These can be diagnosed with modern technology. No other organ, besides the kidney, has been found to have such devastating effect on the whole body. Starve the kidneys of oxygen and they in turn will destroy the brain and heart with hypertension. Fortunately, cases with a "kinked" renal artery are rare. However, Dr. H. Goldblatt, with his research, made a paramount discovery: Oxygen starvation of kidneys causes hypertension and **premature death** *(2)* — **if untreated** *(1)*.

In Dr. Goldblatt's concept, the damaged kidneys cause hypertension. However, such arterial abnormality of the kidneys are relatively rare. What about all the many other patients who suffer with high blood pressure? What could be the reason? In Dr. Goldblatt's concept, the fresh blood loaded with oxygen is not reaching the kidneys because of an obstructive "kink" in the renal artery. There is another more common abnormality in the body, where the kidneys are also deprived of their normal supply of oxygen. In fact, I believe it is the most common cause of high blood pressure. When the blood has given off its oxygen to the kidney cells, and is ready to return to the heart and lungs for another load of oxygen, it meets a resistance on its return flow to the heart. With such impediment to the return flow, the kidney cells again suffer with hypoxia, exactly as in Dr. Goldblatt's patients. Also, with the same general effect, the victim gets general high blood pressure. How is this possible? Where is the return venous flow obstructed?

Normally the renal veins channel the used blood from the kidneys into the **vena cava**. This is the largest vein of the body. It rests in front and along the spine, extending from the pelvis to the heart. Before entering the heart, the vein passes through the back portion of the liver. The "caval canal" in the liver is about 2-3

136

inches long. The liver tissue encircles this venous canal completely, or almost so. A vertebrae of the spine makes the encircling complete. In other words, the liver tissue together with the vertebrae form a 2-3-inches long canal for this large vein. As we know, the liver enlarges during an anaphylactic reaction. As part of this liver enlargement, the canal that contains this large vein is narrowed. Such obstructive narrowing of the liver "canal" has been demonstrated with venograms *(1-15)*. To overcome the liver obstruction resulting from the canal narrowing, requires increased propulsion of the blood. Certain abdominal exercises could help to overcome this stagnant blood circulation of the kidneys.

This resistance to the return blood flow is transmitted from the vena cava to the renal (kidney) veins. This prevents the blood from speedily returning to the heart and lungs for the much needed oxygen. Because of this obstruction to flow, the kidney cells again are damaged with hypoxia. As expected, such suffering kidney cells, also release the same chemicals as renin and angiotensin to flood the whole body. They furthermore cause a salt retension, and a general **artioler** spasm. The total effect is high blood pressure. The cause and effect are similar to Dr. Goldblatt's cases: hypoxia of kidneys by either mechanism results in hypertension, soon requiring a doctor's attention.

Such periods of hypertension may at first be intermittent. For instance, high blood pressure may follow a heavy dinner to which the liver cells have been sensitized. The following days when a more suitable diet is used, the blood pressure returns to normal. However, with repeated anaphylactic reactions to food, the narrowing of the **caval canal** in the liver can become more rigid. A more firm constriction of the caval vein passage, through the liver develops. This causes a continued hypoxin of the kidneys and finally results in a permanent hypertension. We conclude then that the liver is the primary cause of such kidney damage. Therefore, the liver requires the first attention for treatment, to ensure normal kidney function, which in turn will assure a normal blood pressure.

The question now arises, why do not all who follow a general American diet have high blood pressure? And how can such tendency to hypertension be inherited? As we know, hypertension follows in certain families. The father or mother suffered with high blood pressure, and several of the children have the same problem. Such inherited inclination could be explained on the basis of a similar caval vein-liver relation. The passage of the caval vein through the back of the liver is variable. In some individuals the liver tissue encircles the vein entirely; in others, the caval vein is more free and not pressed upon even by an enlarging liver. Close relatives are formed alike. For that family tree, the relation of the caval vein to the liver would be similar. If the caval vein happened to be encircled by a 2-3 inch grasp of liver tissue, an anaphylactic enlargement could impede the return flow of blood to the heart. The final result would be general hypertension.

On the other hand, if the caval vein was relatively free of liver tissue or possibly limited to one side of the caval vein only, such individuals would enjoy a normal blood pressure unaffected by the food they used. Even if the liver enlarged with an allergic reaction, it has no constricting grip on the caval vein.

We can then conclude from this concept that the anaphylactically reacting liver is the main cause of hypertension. Therefore, our treatment must concentrate on the liver. Certain food we eat causes an allergic reaction and results in high blood pressure. Clinically this has been confirmed frequently by vegetarian societies throughout the world. They are too numerous to mention here. Any bookstore has volumes that confirm this fact.

In Brief

At first animal proteins should be reduced to under 50 grams daily, in the form of milk, cheese and eggs. The amount of fats or egg yolk would be determined by the doctor who would, of course, first check the blood cholesterol reading. Only fats and proteins have to be restricted. Carbohydrates (cereals, fruits, vegetables and nuts), usually do not affect the blood pressure. Such dietetic attempts should be undertaken with the close cooperation of the family physician. He would record the diet and the effect on the blood pressure. The full effect on blood pressure with such a controlled diet, appears within four to six weeks. Many patients in such time will enjoy a completely normal blood pressure. Only relatively few, the doctor will find, require a much reduced medical control.

A note of warning should be added here. If the blood pressure has returned to normal for some time, even one dinner with meat can raise the blood pressure to the previous high level. If the patient's blood pressure has been controlled with this special diet, he or she should hold to it for six months. Later, if the patient wants to find his or her tolerance of heavier food, it should be one kind at a time. For instance, at first, small helpings of either **fresh** fish or fowl. If the blood pressure remains unchanged — larger helpings and other meats can be tried. In my experience the portion of meats allowed is very restricted for a controlled hypertensive.

Conclusion

The food we eat causes hypertension. A careless, full diet in many individuals causes kidney hypoxemia. Such damaged kidney tissue releases chemicals into the general circulation which cause general hypertension. The hypertensive patient can reduce the blood pressure by eating certain food which does not cause anaphylactic reactions of the liver, allowing normal blood circulation of the kidneys and normalizing the blood pressure.

References

1. Goldblatt, Harry M.D. et al.: Studies on Experimental Hypertension, J. Experimental Medicine, Vol. 59: 347, 1933
2. Baxter, J. H. and Ashworth, C. T.: Renal Lesions In Portal Cirrhosis, Archives of Pathology, Vol. 46: 476, 1946
3. Baldus, W. P. et al.: Renal Circulation in Cirrhosis: Observations Based on Catheterization of the Renal Vein, J. of Clinical Investigation, Vol. 43: 1090, 1964
4. Lancestremere, Ruben G. et al.: Renal Failure in Laennec's Cirrhosis, J. of Clinical Investigation, Vol. 41: 1922, 1962
5. Mullane, John F. and Gliedman, Marvin L.: Elevation of the Pressure in the Abdominal Inferior Cava as a Cause of Hepatorenal Syndrome in Cirrhosis, Surgery, Vol. 59: 1135, 1966
6. Baldus, W. P. et al.: Renal Circulation in Cirrhosis: Observation Based on Catheterization of the Renal Vein, J. of Clinical Investigation, Vol. 43: 1090, 1964

7. Solomon, Papper, M.D.: Hepatorenal Syndrome, Contr. Nephrology, Vol. 23, pp. 55-74 (Karger, Basel 1980)
8. Salomon, Mardoqueo, M.D., et al.: Renal Lesions in Hepatic Disease, Arch. Internal Medicine, Vol. 115: 704, 1965
9. Gliedman, Marvin L. M.D., et al.: Hepatic Swelling and Inferior Vena Cava Constriction, Annals of Surgery, Vol. 161: 344, 1965
10. Petersen, O. M.D. et al.: Roentgen Examination of the Inferior Vena Cava in Chronic Hepatic Disease, Acta Radiologica, Vol. 55: 97, 1960
11. Huddle, K. R.: Amoebic Liver Abscess, Inferior Vena-Caval Compression and the Nephrotic Syndrome, S.A. Medical Journal, May 15, 1982
12. Wilkinson, S. P., et al.: Spectrum of Renal Tubular Damage in Renal Failure Secondary to Cirrhosis and Fulminant Hepatic Failure, J. of Clinical Pathology, Vol. 31, pp. 101-107, 1978
13. Selkurt, Ewald E., et al.: Response of Renal Blood Flow and Clearance to Graded Partial Obstruction of the Renal Vein, Am. J. Physiology, Vol. 157, pp. 40-46, 1949
14. Bell, E. T., et al.: The Causes of Hypertension, Am. Int. Med., Vol. 4, pp. 227-239, 1930/31
15. Pedersen, A. H.: A Method of Producing Experimental Chronic Hypertension in the Rabbit, Arch. of Pathology and Laboratory Medicine, Vol. 3, p. 912, 1927

Other References

1. Martin, Arthur M. and Hackel, Donald B.: The Myocardium of the Dog in Hemorrhagic Shock, Laboratory Investigation, Vol. 12: 77, 1963.
2. Melcher, George W. and Walcott, William W.: Myocardial Changes Following Shock, American Journal of Physiology, Vol. 164 (3): 832, 1951.
3. Martin, Arthur M. et al.: Human Myocardial Zonal Lesions, Arch. Pathol., Vol. 87: 339, 1969.
4. Whaley, Robert L. et al.: Hemodynamic and Myocardial Changes in Anaphylactic Shock, Circulation, Vol. 28: 826, 1963.
4.(a) Eliot, Robert S. M.D., Salhany, Emily A. B.S., R.D.: Sudden Death and Acute Myocardial Infarction, Post Graduate Medicine, Vol. 64, #4, 52, Oct./78.
5. Delage, Claude et al.: Myocardial Lesions in Anaphylaxis, Arch. Pathol., Vol. 95: 185, 1973.
6. Martin, Arthur M. et al.: The Ultrastructure of Zonal Lesions of the Myocardium in Hemorrhagic Shock, Am. J. of Pathology, Vol. 44: 127, Jan. 1964.
7. Martin, Arthur M. et al.: Mechanisms in the Development of Myocardial Lesions in Hemorrhagic Shock, Annals New York Academy of Sciences, Vol. 156: 79, Jan. 1969.

8.   Nishimura, E. T. et al.: Myocardial Lesions Associated with Experimental Passive Transfer of Immediate Type Hypersensitivity, Laboratory Investigation, Vol. 15: 1269, 1966.

9.   McManus, J. F. and Lawlor, J. J.: Myocardial Infarction Following the Administration of Tetanus Antitoxin, The New England Journal of Medicine, Vol. 242: 17, 1950.

10.   Hackel, D. B. et al.: Hemorrhagic Shock in Dogs, Archives of Pathology, Vol. 77: 575, 1964.

11.   Wadsworth, G. H. and Brown, C. H.: Serum Reaction Complicated by Acute Carditis, The Journal of Pediatrics, Vol. 17: 801, 1940.

12.   Entman, Mark L. et al.: Phasic Myocardial Blood Flow in Hemorrhagic Hypotension, Am. J. of Cardiology, Vol. 21: 881, 1968.

13.   Henschen, C.: Die Akuten, Subakuten un Chronischen Schwellungskrisen der Leber (Akutes und Chronisches Leberglaukom) und ihr Chirurgische Behandlung, Archiv. Fur Klinische Chirurgie, Vol. 167: 825, 1931.

14.   Reich, Theobald: Hepatoportal Circulation and its Clinical Implications, New York State Journal of Medicine, p. 947, May 1, 1971.

14.(a) Knisely, Melvin H. et al.: Hepatic Sphincters, Science, Vol. 125: 1023, 1957.

15.   McCuskey, Robert S.: A Dynamic and Static Study of Hepatic Arterioles and Hepatic Sphincters, Am. J. Anat., Vol. 119: 455.

16.   Andrews, W. H. Horner et al.: Studies of the Liver Circulation, Ann. Trop. Med. Parasit., Vol. 43: 229, Oct. 1949.

17.   Deysach, L. J.: The Nature and Location of the "Sphincter Mechanism" in the Liver as Determined by Drug Actions and Vascular Injections, American Journal of Physiology, Vol. 132: 713, 1941.

18.   Snyder, Charles D.: Some Vascular Responses Within the Liver and Their Interpretation, Rev. of Gastroent., Vol. 9: 230, 1942.

19.   Seneviratne, R. D.: Physiological and Ethological Responses in the Blood Vessels of the Liver, Quarterly J. of Experimental Physiology, Vol. 35: 6, 1949.

20.   Blalock, Alfred and Mason, Morton F.: Observations on the Blood Flow and Gaseous Metabolism of the Liver of Unanesthetized Dogs, Am. J. Physiology, Vol. 117: 328, 1936

21.   Bolton, Charles and Barnard, W. G.: The Pathological Occurrences in the Liver in Experimental Venous Stagnation, Journ. of Path., Vol. XXXIV: 701, 1931.

22.   Pribram, B. O.: Ueber Passive Leberzellgymnastik, Munch. Med. Wschr., Nr. 49: 1993, Dec. 1936.

23.   Voegtlin, Carl and Bernheim, B. M.: The Liver in its Relation to Anaphylactic Shock, Journal of Pharmacology and Ex-

perimental Therapeutics, Vol. 2: 507, 1910/11.
24. Weil, Richard: Studies in Anaphylaxis, Journal of Immunology, Vol. 2: 109, 1916/17.
25. Weil, Richard: The Vasomotor Depression in Canine Anaphylaxis, Journal of Immunology, Vol. 2: 429, 1916/17.
26. Weil, Richard: Studies in Anaphylaxis, Journal of Immunology, Vol. 2: 525, 1917.
27. Manwaring, W. H. et al.: Hepatic Reactions in Anaphylaxis, Journal of Immun., Vol. 8: 121, 1922.
28. Manwaring, W. H. and Boyd, Walter H.: Hepatic Reactions in Anaphylaxis, Journal of Immun., Vol. 8: 131, 1922.
29. Selkurt, Ewald E.: Role of Liver and Toxic Factors in Shock, Anesth. Clin., Vol. 2: 201-221, Feb. 1964.
30. Manwaring, W. H. et al.: Hepatic Reactions in Anaphylaxis, Journal of Immun., Vol. 8: 191, 1922.
31 Manwaring, W. H. et al.: Hepatic Reactions in Anaphylaxis, Journal of Immun., Vol. 8: 217, 1923.
32. Manwaring, W. H. et al.: Hepatic Reactions in Anaphylaxis, Journal of Immun., Vol. 8: 229, 1923.
33. Manwaring, W. H. et al.: Hepatic Reactions in Anaphylaxis, Journal of Immun., Vol. 8: 233, 1923.
34. Simonds, J. P. and Brandes, W. W.: The Effect of Mechanical Obstruction of the Hepatic Veins Upon the Outflow of Lymph From the Thoracic Duct, Journal of Immun., Vol. 13: 11, 1926.
35. Simonds, J. P. and Brandes W. W.: Anaphylactic Shock and Mechanical Obstruction of the Hepatic Veins in the Dog, Journal of Immun., Vol. 13: 1, 1926.
36. Weatherford, Harold L.: The Influence of Anaphylactic Shock on the Finer Structure of the Liver in the Dog, Am. J. Path., Vol. 11: 611, 1935.
37. MacLean, L. D. et al.: Canine Intestinal and Liver Weight Changes Induced by E. Coli Endotoxin, Proc. Soc. Exp. Biol. and Med., Vol. 92: 602, 1956.
38. Shoemaker, William C. et al.: Hepatic Hemodynamic and Morphologic Changes in Shock, Arch. Path., Vol. 80: 76, 1965.
39. Glynn, L. E. and Himsworth, H. P.: The Intralobular Circulation in Acute Liver Injury by Carbon Tetrachloride, J. Clin. Sci., Vol. 6: 235, 1946.
40. Manwaring, W. H. et al.: Hepatic Reactions in Anaphylaxis, Journal of Immun., Vol. 8: 211, 1923.
41. Louros, N.: Zur Pathologie der Leber bei der Anaphylaxie, Arch. Exp. Path., Vol. 121: 238, 1927.
42. Bywaters, E. G. L.: Anatomical Changes in the Liver After Trauma, Clinical Science, Vol. 6: 19, 1947.
43. Hartley, G. and Lushbaugh, C. C.: Experimental Allergic Focal Necrosis of the Liver, Am. J. Path., Vol. 18: 1942.

44. Denecke, Gerhard: Uber die Bedeutung der Leber fur die Anaphylaktische Reaktion beim Hunde, Zeitschr. F. Immunitatsforschung, Vol. 20: 501, 1913.

45. Shamberger, Raymond J. et al.: Malonaldehyde Content of Food, Journal of Nutrition, Vol. 107: 1404, 1977.

46. Brooks, B. R. and Klamerth, O. L.: Interaction of DNA with Bifunctional Aldehydes, European Journal Biochem. Vol. 5: 178, 1968.

47. Schaffner, Fenton et. al: Hepatic Mesenchymal Cell Reaction in Liver Disease, Exper. and Molec. Path., Vol. 2: 419, 1962.

48. Bloch, Edward H.: The In Vivo Microscopic Vascular Anatomy and Physiology of the Liver as Determined with the Quartz Rod Method of Transillumination, Angiology, Vol. 6: 340-349, 1955.

49. Friedberg, Charles: Diseases of the Heart, p. 775, W. B. Saunders Co.

49.(a) Russel, Jane A.: Biochemical Studies.

50. Holroyde, C. and Eyre, Peter: Enterohepatic Haemodynamics in Calves During Acute Systemic Anaphylaxis, European J. Pharmac., Vol. 30: 43, 1975.

51. MacLean, Lloyd D. et al.: Hypotension (Shock) in Dogs Produced by Escherichia Coli Endotoxin, Circulation Research, Vol. 4: 546, 1956.

52. Voegtlin, Carl and Bernheim, B. M.: The Liver in its Relation to Anaphylactic Shock, J. Pharm. Exp. Ther., Vol. 2: 507, 1910.

53. Petersen, William F. et al.: Studies in Endothelial Permeability, Journal of Immuno., Vol. 8: 361, 1923.

54. Petersen, William F. et al.: Studies on Endothelial Permeability, Journal of Immuno., Vol. 8: 367, 1923.

55. Barret, J. T.: The Immediate or Immunoglobulin-Dependent Hypersensitivities, Text Book of Immun., p. 255, 1974.

56. Andrews, W. H. Horner and Maegraith, B. G.: The Pathogenesis of the Liver Lesion Due to the Administration of Carbon Tetrachloride, Ann. Trop. Med. Parasit., Vol. 42: 95, 1948.

57. Frank, Howard, A. et. al: Traumatic Shock. XIII. The Prevention of Irreversibility in Hemorrhagic Shock by Vivi-perfusion of the Liver, Journal Clinical Investigation, Vol. 25: 22, 1946.

58. Buis, L. James and Hartman, F. W.: Histopathology of the Liver Following Superficial Burns, Am. J. Clin. Path., Vol. 11: 275-287, April, 1941.

59. Rosenmund, A.: Ein Leberspezifisches Antigen im Serum von Leberkranken, Schweiz. Med. Wschr., Vol. 101: 1023, 1971.

60. Anlyan, William G. et al.: A Study of Liver Damage Following Induced Hypotension, Surgery, Vol. 36: 375, 1954.

61. Dean, H. R.: The Histology of a Case of Anaphylactic Shock

Occuring in a Man, J. Path. and Bacteriology, Vol. 25: 305, 1922.

62. Gurd, Fraser B. and Emrys-Roberts, E.: Fatal Anaphylaxis, The Lancet, p. 763, April 3, 1920.

63. Murphy, E. S. and Mireles, Mario: Shock, Liver Necrosis, and Death After Penicillin Injection, Archives of Pathology, Vol. 73: 355, 1963.

64. Wilson, W. C. et al.: The Clinical Course and Pathology of Burns and Scalds Under Modern Methods of Treatment, British J. of Surgery, Vol. 25: 826, April, 1938.

65. Dean, H. R. and Webb, R. A.: The Morbid Anatomy and Histology of Anaphylaxis in the Dog, J. of Path. and Bacteriology, Vol. 27: 51, 1924.

66. Blanton, W. B.: Anaphylaxis Due to Stinging Insects, Occupational Medicine, Vol. 9: 87, 1967.

67. Hanashiro, Paul K. and Weil, M. H.: Anaphylactic Shock in Man, Arch. Int. Med., Vol. 119: 129, 1967.

68. Glynn, L. E. and Himsworth, H. P.: The Intralobular Circulation in Acute Liver Injury by Carbon Tetrachloride, Clin. Science, Vol. 67: 235, 1946.

69. Peters, Gustavus A. et al.: Anaphylactic Penicillin Reactions: Three Non-fatal Cases of Reaction to Oral Penicillin with Positive Skin Tests and One Fatal Case following Intramuscular Penicillin, Staff Meetings of the Mayo Clinic, Vol. 30: 634, 1955.

70. Maganzini, Herman C.: Anaphylactoid Reaction to Penicillins V and G Administered Orally, New Eng. J. Med., Vol. 256: 52, 1957.

71. Hardaway, Robert M. et al.: Studies on the Role of Intravascular Coagulation in Irreversible Hemorrhagic Shock, Annals of Surgery, Vol. 155: 241, 1962.

72. Hardaway, Robert M. and Johnson, D. G.: Influence of Fibrinolysin on Shock, J.A.M.A., Vol. 183: 177, 1963.

73. Ettinger, M. G.: Coagulation Studies in Cerebrovascular Disease, Neurology, Vol. 14: 907, 1964.

74. Todd, Margaret et al.: Stroke and Blood Coagulation, Stroke, Vol. 4: 400, 1973.

75. Wu, Kenneth K. and Hoak, John C.: Increased Platelet Aggregates in Patients with Transient Ischemic Attacks, Stroke, Vol. 6: 521, 1975.

76. Davis, James W.: Defective Platelet Disaggregation Associated with Occlusive Arterial Diseases, Angiology, Vol. 24: 391, 1973.

77. Hardaway, Robert M.: The Role of Intravascular Clotting in the Etiology of Shock, Annals of Surgery, Vol. 155: 325, 1962.

78. McIver, M. A. et al.: Gaseous Exchange Between the Blood

145

and the Lumen of Stomach and Intestine, Am. J. of Physiology, Vol. 76: 92, 1926.

79. Olson, E. G. T.: Myocardial Infarction, Chap. 5, p. 47, The Pathology of the Heart.

80. Baroldi, Giorgio et al.: Sudden Coronary Death. A Postmortem Study, Am. Heart J., Vol. 98: 20, 1979.

81. Baroldi, Giorgio, M.D., Robert S. Eliot, M.D.: The Pathophysiology of Coronary Heart Disease Contemp. Probs in Cardiology, 3: 1, 1977.

82. Spain, David M. et al.: Sudden Death from Coronary Heart Disease, Chest, 58: 107, 1970.

83. Baroldi, Giorgio: Different Types of Myocardial Necrosis in Coronary Heart Disease: A Pathophysiologic Review of their Functional Significance, Am. Heart Journal, 89: 742, 1975.

84. Lie, J. T., M.D., and Titus, J. L.: Pathology of the Myocardium and the Conduction System in Sudden Heart Death, Circulation Suppl. 3, Vol. 51: 41, 1975.

85. Pitt, Berthram, M.D. et al.: Myocardial Imaging in the Noninvasive Evaluation of Patients with Suspected Ischemic Heart Disease, The Am. J. of Cardiology, 37: 797, 1976.

86. Baroldi, G. et al.: Significance of Morphological Changes in Sudden Coronary Death, Adv. Cardiol, Vol. 25: 82 (Karger, Basel, 1978).

87. Eliot, R. S. et al.: Necropsy Studies in Myocardial Infarction with Minimal or No Luminal Reduction Due to Atherosclerosis Circulation, 49: 1127, 1974.

88. Baroldi, Giorgio, M.D.: Coronary Heart Disease: Significance of the Morphologic Lesions, Am. Heart J., Vol. 85: 1, 1973.

89. Silver, Malcolm, D., M.D., PH.D. et al.: The Relationship Between Acute Occlusive Coronary Thrombi and Myocardial Infarction Studied in 100 Consecutive Patients, An Official J. of the Am. Heart Assoc. Inc., Vol. 61: 219, 1980.

90. Baroldi, Giorgio, M.D.: Coronary Thrombosis: Facts and Beliefs Am. Heart J., Vol. 91: 683, 1976.

91. Baroldi, Giorgio, M.D.: Coronary Stenosis: Ischemic or non-ischemic factor? Am. Heart J., Vol. 96: 139, 1978.

92. Baroldi, G. et al.: Morphology of Acute Myocardial Infarction in Relation to Coronary Thrombosis, Am. Heart J., Vol. 87: 65, 1974.

93. Friedman, Meyer, M.D. et. al: Instantaneous and Sudden Deaths Clinical and Pathological Differentiation of Coronary Artery Disease, J.A.M.A. 225: 1319, 1973.

94. Chandler, A. B. et al.: Coronary Thrombosis in Myocardial Infarction, The Am. J. or Cardiology, Vol. 34: 823, 1974.

95. Spain, D. M.: The Pathogenesis of Sudden Cardiac Death and the Sequelae of Myocardial Infarction, The Heart, p. 67.

96. Bouchardy, B. and Majno, G.: Histopathology of Early Myocardial Infarcts, Am. J. of Path., Vol. 74: 301, 1974.

97. Riesman, D. and Harris, S. E.: Disease of the Coronary Arteries with a Consideration of Data on the Increasing Mortality of Heart Disease, Am. J. Med. Sciences, Jan. 1934.

98. Lucas, B. G. B.: Role of Anoxia and Hypoxia in Etiology of Cardiac Arrest, Cardiac Arrest and Resuscitation, Fourth Edition, p. 166.

99. Baroldi, G. et al.: Sudden Coronary Death: A Postmortem Study in 208 Selected Cases Compared to 97 "Control" Subjects, Am. Heart Journal, Vol. 98: 20, 1979.

100. Haerem, J. W.: Mural Platelet Microthrombi and Major Acute Lesions of Main Epicardial Arteries in Sudden Coronary Death, Atherosclerosis, Vol. 19: 529, 1974.

101. Shubin, H. and Weil, M. H.: Acute Elevation of Serum Transaminase and Lactic Dehydrogenase During Circulatory Shock, Am. J. of Card., p. 327, March, 1963.

102. Alonso, D. R. et al.: Early Quantification of Experimental Myocardial Infarction with Technetium-99m Glucoheptonate: Scintigraphic and Anatomic Studies, Am. J. of Card., Vol. 42: 251, August, 1978.

103. Spector, F. and Spain, D. M.: The Pathology of Sudden Death and the Ability to Predicts its Occurrence, Circulation Suppl. II, Vol. 45: 225, October, 1972.

104. Roberts, W. C.: The Coronary Arteries in Fatal Coronary Events, Controversy in Cardiology, Chapter 1, p. 1.

105. Lie, J. T. et al.: Morphological Evidence of Myocardial Ischemia in Sudden, Unexpected Death from Coronary Heart Disease, Circulation Suppl. II, Vol. 43: 45, 1971.

106. Page, D. L. et al.: Myocardial Changes Associated with Cardiogenic Shock, New Eng. J. Med., Vol. 285: 133, 1971.

107. Eliot, R. S. et al.: Necropsy Studies in Myocardial Infarction with Minimal or No Coronary Luminal Reduction Due to Atherosclerosis, Circulation, Vol. 49: 1127, 1974.

108. Miller, R. D. et al.: Myocardial Infarction With and Without Acute Coronary Occlusion, A.M.A. Arch. of Int. Med., Vol. 88: 597, 1951.

109. Parkey, R. W. et al.: A New Method for Radionuclide Imaging of Acute Myocardial Infarction in Humans, Circulation, Vol. 50: 540, 1974.

110. Moritz, A. R. and Zamcheck, N.: Sudden and Unexpected Deaths of Young Soldiers, Archives of Path., Vol. 42: 459, 1946.

111. Weisberger, C. L. et al.: Treatment of Cardiogenic Shock, Controversy in Cardiology, Chapter 5, p. 67.

112. Shoemaker, W. C.: Shock: Chemistry, Physiology and Therapy, Shock, p. 78.

113. Osler, W.: Angina Pectoris, The Lancet, p. 697, March 12, 1910, p. 839, March 26, 1910, p. 973, April 9, 1910.
114. Eliot, R. S. et al.: Influence of Environmental Stress of Pathogenesis of Sudden Cardiac Death, Federation Proceedings, Vol. 36: 1719, 1977.
115. Perper, J. A. et al.: Arteriosclerosis of Coronary Arteries in Sudden, Unexpected Deaths, Circulation Suppl. III, Vol. 51: 27, 1975.
116. Roma, M.: II Review of the Literature, Acta Medica Scandinavica Suppl. 547, 1972.
117. Friedberg, C.: Acute Coronary Occlusion and Myocardial Infarction, Diseases of the Heart, p. 775.
118. Wolff, L. and White, P. D.: Acute Coronary Occlusion, Boston Med. and Surg. J., Vol. 195: 13, 1926.
119. Phipps, C.: Contributory Causes of Coronary Thrombosis, J.A.M.A., Vol. 106: 761, 1936.
120. Master, A. M. et al.: Factors and Events Asociated with Onset of Coronary Artery Thrombosis, J.A.M.A., Vol. 109: 546, 1937.
121. Luten, D.: Contributory Factors in Coronary Occlusion, Am. Heart Journal, Vol. 7: 36, 1931.
122. Hardaway, Robert M. et al.: Endotoxin Shock, Annals of Surgery, Vol. 154: 791, 1961.
123. Leonhardt, H. and Bungert, H. J.: Rheologische Untersuchungen bei der Chronisch-aggressiven Hepatitis, Zeitschrift fur Gastroenterologie, Vol. 6: 588, 1975.
124. Levenson, Stanley M. et al.: Some Metabolic Consequences of Shock, International Anes. Clinic, Vol. 2: 237, 1964.
125. Pirkle, Hubert: Pulmonary Platelet Aggregates Associated with Sudden Death in Man, Science, Vol. 185: 1062, 1974.
126. Pilgeram, L. O.: Abnormalities in Clotting and Thrombolysis as a Risk Factor for Stroke, Thrombos. Diathes. Haemorrh. (Stuttg.), Vol. 31: 245, 1974.
127. Hardaway, Robert M. et al.: Studies on the Role of Intravascular Coagulation in Irreversible Haemorrhagic Shock, Annals of Surgery, Vol. 155: 241, 1962.
128. Hardaway, Robert M. et al.: The Role of Intravascular Clotting in the Etiology of Shock, Annals of Surgery, Vol. 155: 325, 1962.
129. The Systemic Response to Shock, Shock A.P. Thal., p. 49, 1971.
130. Kerp, L. and Kasemir, H.: Der Immunologisch Ausgeloste Schock, Med. Welt, Vol. 22: 1166, 1971.
131. Shoemaker, William C.: Hepatic Microcirculatory Changes in Shock, Shock: Chemistry, Physiology and Therapy, p. 48-55.
132. Eckstein, R. W.: Effect of Exercise and Coronary Artery Narrowing on Coronary Collateral Circulation, Circulation

Research, Vol. 5: 230, 1957.
133. Morris, J. N. and Crawford, M. D.: Coronary Heart Disease and Physical Activity of Work, British Med. J., Dec. 20, 1958.
134. Fox III, Samuel M. et al.: Physical Activity and Coronary Heart Disease, Physical Fitness Research Digest, Series 2, No. 2, April, 1972.
135. Lopez-s, A. et al.: Effect of Exercise and Physical Fitness on Serum Lipids and Lipoproteins, Atherosclerosis, Vol. 20:, 1, 1974.
136. Hanson, J. S. and Neede, W. H.: Preliminary Observations on Physical Training for Hypertensive Males, Circulation Research, Vol. 26: 1-49, 1970.
137. Mann, George V. et al.: Physical Fitness and Immunity to Heart-Disease in Masai, The Lancet, p. 1308, Dec. 25, 1965.
138. Frank, Charles W. et al.: Physical Inactivity as a Lethal Factor in Myocardial Infarction Among Men, Circulation, Vol. 34: 1022, 1966.
139. Carlstrom, S. and Karlefors, T.: Plasma-Free-Fatty-Acids in Diabetics During Exercise, The Lancet, Feb. 8, 1964.
140. Fox III, S. M. et al.: Physical Activity and Cardiovascular Health, Modern Concepts of Cardiovascular Disease, Vol. 41: 17, 1972.
141. Letters to the Editor: Exercise and Blood-Fibrinolysis, The Lancet, Nov. 26, 1966.
142. Pomeroy, W. C. et al.: Coronary Heart Disease in Former Football Players, J.A.M.A., Vol. 167: 711, 1958.
143. Taylor, H. L. et al.: Death Rates Among Physically Active and Sedentary Employees of the Railroad Industry, A.J.P.H., Vol. 52: 1697, Oct. 1962.
144. Laurie, W.: Prevention of Myocardial Infarction, The Med. J. of Australia, p. 361, Feb. 13, 1971.
145. Menon, I. S. et al.: Effect of Strenuous and Graded Exercise on Fibrinolytic Activity, The Lancet, April 1, 1967.
146. Motta, J. A. et al.: Submaximal Exercise Testing in a Random and High Lipid Samples from Three Northern California Communities, Circulation Suppl. III, Vol. 49: 111-115, Oct. 1974.
147. Jokl, Ernst: Exercise and Cardiac Death, J.A.M.A., Vol. 218: 1707, 1971.
148. Mann, George V. et al.: The Amount of Exercise Necessary to Achieve and Maintain Fitness in Adult Persons, Southern Med. J., Vol. 64: 549, May, 1971.
149. Ganong, W. F.: Review of Medical Physiology, Lange Pub., Seventh Edition, p. 464.
150. Taylor, C. B. et al.: Spontaneously Occurring Angiotoxic Derivatives of Cholesterol, The Am. J. Clin. Nutrition, Vol. 32: 40, 1979.

151. Mukai, F. H. and Goldstein, B. D.: Mutagenicity of Malonaldehyde, a Decomposition Product of Peroxidized Polyunsaturated Fatty Acids, Science, Vol. 191: 869, 1976.

152. Bidlack, Wayne R. et al.: Production and Binding of Malonaldehyde During Storage of Cooked Pork, Journal of Food Science, Vol. 37: 664, 1972.

153. Siu, G. M. and Draper, H. H.: A Survey of the Malonaldehyde Content of Retail Meats and Fish, Journal of Food Science, Vol. 43: 1147, 1978.

154. Klamerth, O. L. and Levinsky, H.: Template Activity in Liver DNA from Rats Fed with Malondialdehyhde, Febs Letters, Vol. 3: 205, 1969, (North Holland Pub. Co., Amsterdam).

155. Guyton, Arthur C., M.D.: Textbook of Medical Physiology, 5th Edition, W. B. Saunders Co., Toronto.

156. McArdle, William D., Katch, Frank I., Katch, Victor L.: Exercise Physiology.

157. Lea and Ferbinger, 1981: Review of Medical Physiology, 7th Edition, Lange Medical Publications.

158. Goldblatt, Harry M. D. et al.: Studies on Experimental Hypertension, J. Experimental Medicine, Vol. 59: 347, 1933.

159. Baxter, J. H. and Ashworth, C. T.: Renal Lesions in Portal Cirrhosis, Archives of Pathology, Vol. 46: 476, 1946.

160. Baldus, W. P. et al.: Renal Circulation in Cirrhosis: Observations Based on Catheterization of the Renal Vein, J. of Clinical Investigation, Vol. 43: 1090, 1964.

161. Lancestremere, Ruben G. et al.: Renal Failure in Laennec's Cirrhosis, J. of Clinical Investigation, Vol. 41: 1922, 1962.

162. Mullane, John F. and Gliedman, Marvin L.: Elevation of the Pressure in the Abdominal Inferior Cava as a Cause of a Hepatorenal Syndrome in Cirrhosis, Surgery, Vol. 59: 1135, 1966.

163. Baldus, W. P. et al.: Renal Circulation in Cirrhosis: Observation Based on Catheterization of the Renal Vein, J. of Clinical Investigation, Vol. 43: 1090, 1964.

164. Solomon, Papper, M.D.: Hepatorenal Syndrome, Contr. Nephrology, Vol. 23: 55-74 (Karger, Basel 1980)

165. Salomon, Mardoqueo, M.D. et al.: Renal Lesions in Hepatic Disease, Arch. Internal Medicine, Vol. 115: 704, 1965.

166. Gliedman, Marvin L., M.D. et al.: Hepatic Swelling and Inferior Vena Cava Constriction, Annals of Surgery, Vol. 161: 344, 1965.

167. Petersen, O., M.D. et al.: Roentgen Examination of the Inferior Vena Cava in Chronic Hepatic Disease, Acta Radiologica, Vol. 55: 97, 1960.

168. Huddle, K. R.: Amoebic Liver Abscess, Inferior Vena-Caval

Compression and the Nephrotic Syndrome, S. A. Medical Journal, May 15, 1982.

169.   Wilkinson, S. P. et al.: Spectrum of Renal Tubular Damage in Renal Failure Secondary to Cirrhosis and Fulminant Hepatic Failure, J. of Clinical Pathology, Vol. 31: 101-107, 1978.

170.   Selkurt, Ewald E. et al.: Response of Renal Blood Flow and Clearance to Graded Partial Obstruction of the Renal Vein, Am. J. Physiology, Vol. 157: 40-46, 194.

171.   Bell, E. T. et al.: The Causes of Hypertension, Am. Int. Med., Vol. 4: 227-239, 1930/31.

172.   Pedersen, A. H.: A Method of Producing Experimental Chronic Hypertension in the Rabbit, Arch. of Pathology and Laboratory Medicine, Vol. 3: 912, 1927.

GLOSSARY

Allergy: Tissue reaction to a substance.

Anaphylaxis: Involvement of several body organs to an allergic reaction with a circulatory collapse.

Anoxic Blood: Blood carrying less oxygen than it is capable.

Antibody: A class of proteins serving to immunize the body against special antigens.

Antigen: A substance causing an allergic reaction.

Arterial: A blood vessel.

Arteriole: Small artery.

Atherosclerosis: Inner coating and hardening of blood vessels, arteries.

A.V. or S.A. Nodes: Centers in the heart from which contraction or beats of the heart muscle originates.

Bronchial Spasm: Bronchial tubes narrow, due to spasms, as in asthma.

Capillaries: The smallest blood vessels.

Carbohydrates: One food classification, e.g. rice, etc.

Cardiac Arrhythmias: Irregular heart beats.

Caudate Lobe: See illustration — one part of liver.

Caval Canal: A narrow passage for the vein; Vena Cava — back part of the liver.

Central Necrosis: The death of the center of a part. In the liver the cells are arranged in lobules, with each having a center. Death then would be in the center of each lobule.

Cerebrovascular: Blood vessels of the brain.

Cholesterol: A fat produced by the liver. Excess cholesterol can coat the inner lining of arteries.

Coagulation: Blood clotting, that is, becoming a solid from a fluid state.

Coagulative Components:	Chemicals which cause clotting.
Collateral Circulation:	A secondary blood supply route after the main route is blocked.
Conducting Mechanism:	Connection between nodes and heart muscle.
Coronary:	Arteries of the heart muscle.
Denaturization:	Deterioration of fresh meat by exposing meat to cooking then storing it open to action of air.
Detoxifying:	Removing of toxins or poisons.
Diaphragm:	Muscle between the lungs and the abdomen, for filling the lungs with air by its movement.
Edematous:	Pertaining to being swollen with water.
Endotoxin:	A harmful substance made in the body.
Eschar:	Skin or muscle destroyed by heat.
Extra Systoles:	Extra heart beats.
Fibrillation:	Fast and irregular beating of the heart.
Foreign Protein Reaction:	An allergic reaction where degenerated protein is the cause.
Glucose:	A sugar; the food we eat for energy is finally digested to glucose. Every body function depends upon glucose.
Haemorrhagic Shock:	Shock due to excessive bleeding.
Hematocrit:	Blood colour a percentage of cell readings, normal 40-45%.
Hemoconcentration:	Thickening of blood, due to abnormal increase in the number of red blood cells to plasma.
Hemodynamics:	Studying the forces involved in circulating the blood in the body.
Hepatic Artery:	Blood vessel that carries fresh blood to the liver.
Hepatic Vein:	The vein that channels the blood from the liver to the heart.
Hepatic Vein Pressure:	The blood pressure where the blood flow leaves the liver toward the heart.
Hypersensitization:	When body tissues become unusually sensitive allergically.
Hypoglycemia:	Blood sugar which is abnormally low.
Hypoemia:	Insufficient blood.
Hypotension:	Low blood pressure.
Hypothesis:	Theory.
Hypovolemic:	Low volume of blood flow.
Hypoxemia:	Insufficient oxygen in the blood.
Hypoxia:	Insufficient oxygen anywhere in the body.
Hypoxic Hepatosis:	Deterioration of liver cells due to insufficient oxygen supply.
Immunology:	The principle of allergic reaction to antigens.
Infarction:	Dead muscle or tissue due to a cessation of blood supply.

Inferior Vena Cava:	See illustration; large vein carrying blood to heart from lower half of body.
Intrahepatic Pressure:	Blood pressure within the liver mass.
Ischemia:	Insufficient blood to sustain life.
Laryngeal Edema:	The larynx swollen with water.
Lobules:	The smallest unit of liver cells which form the whole liver.
Melonaldehyde:	A chemical produced only in meat due to oxidation (exposure to air).
Metabolic:	The sum of all physical and chemical changes that take place within an organism — the body.
Microcirculatory Collapse:	Closure of the small blood vessels.
Micro-Pathological:	Microscopic description of muscle or any tissue damage.
Morphological:	The structural findings.
Myocardial:	Heart muscle.
Myocardial Deterioration:	Heart muscle damage due to insufficient oxygen, or muscle death.
Myocardial Infarction:	A partial or completely dead portion of a heart muscle, due to insufficient blood supply.
Myocytolysis:	Muscle fiber disintegration.
Myofibers:	Muscle fibers.
Necrotic:	Death of a section of tissue or muscle.
Occlusive Coronary Thrombosis:	Closure of a heart artery due to a blood clot.
Parenterally:	By injection with a needle into body, through the skin.
Pathophysiology:	The physiology of disordered function.
Plasma:	The clear fluid portion of blood.
Portal Hypertension:	High blood pressure in the portal vein, due to obstruction of blood flow through the liver toward the heart.
Portal System:	Veins which collect blood from the abdominal organs and conveys it to the sinusoids of the liver.
Portal Vein:	The main vein that carries the blood from stomach, intestines, spleen and pancreas, to the liver.
Protein Sensitization:	A body tissue sensitization to abnormal proteins before an allergic reaction.
Sinusoids:	Canals in the liver in which the blood flows between the cells.
Sinusoidal Endothelium:	The liver cells which form the sinusoidal canals.
Sphincter:	A circular muscle, which when contracted, closes a canal.
Splanchic Pool:	Full blood vessels of the abdomen.

Stenotic:	Narrowing by atherosclerosis.
Stroke Volume:	The volume of blood the heart pumps with each contraction.
Subendocardial:	Under the lining of the heart cavity.
Subendocardial Coagulative Myocytosis:	Dead heart muscle under the heart lining due to lack of oxygen.
Thrombosis:	Clotting of blood in a blood vessel.
Thrombotic Occlusion:	Artery or vein closed by a clot.
Transmural Coagulative Necrosis:	The death of muscle due to the clotting of blood in the area.
Vasoconstriction:	General narrowing of small arteries (arterioles).
Vena Cava:	Vessel in which blood flows from the legs and lower abdomen to the heart.
Venous:	Blood flowing in a vein from any part of the body, back to the heart.
Venous Blood:	Blood flowing back to the heart in a vein.
Viviperfusion:	Arranging a blood transfusion to the liver, outside of the portal vein and hepatic artery, to a living body.

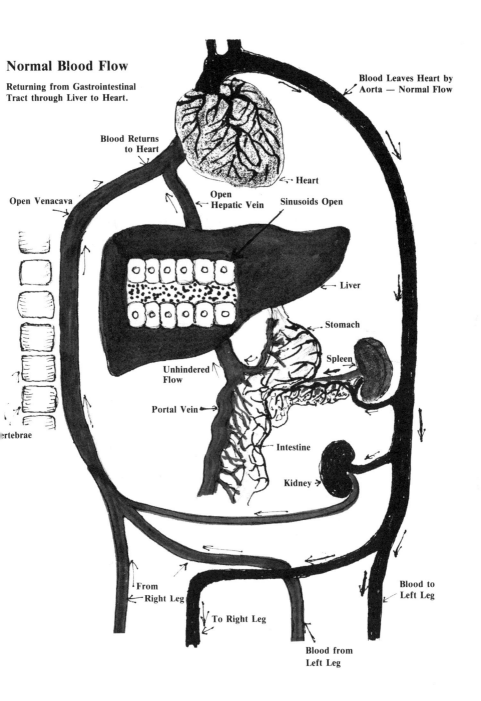

Normal Blood Flow

Returning from Gastrointestinal Tract through Liver to Heart.

Blood Leaves Heart by Aorta — Normal Flow

Blood Returns to Heart

Open Venacava

Open Hepatic Vein

Sinusoids Open

Heart

Liver

Stomach

Spleen

Unhindered Flow

Portal Vein

Intestine

Kidney

Vertebrae

From Right Leg

To Right Leg

Blood to Left Leg

Blood from Left Leg

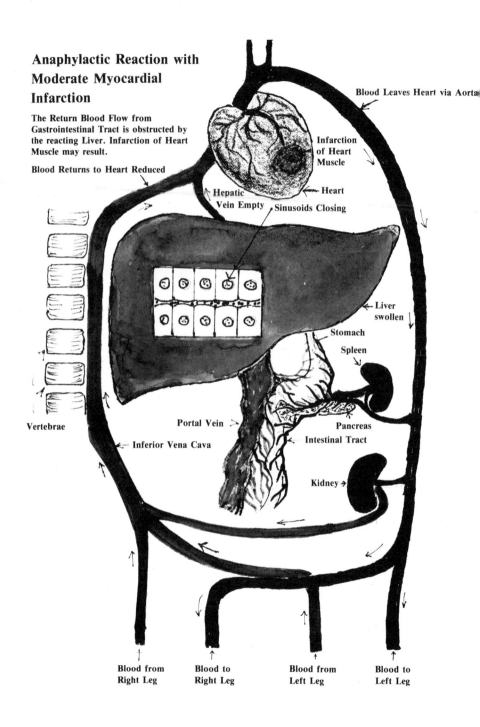

Anaphylactic Reaction with Moderate Myocardial Infarction

The Return Blood Flow from Gastrointestinal Tract is obstructed by the reacting Liver. Infarction of Heart Muscle may result.

Blood Returns to Heart Reduced

Blood Leaves Heart via Aorta

Infarction of Heart Muscle

Hepatic Vein Empty

Heart

Sinusoids Closing

Liver swollen

Stomach

Spleen

Vertebrae

Portal Vein

Inferior Vena Cava

Pancreas

Intestinal Tract

Kidney

Blood from Right Leg

Blood to Right Leg

Blood from Left Leg

Blood to Left Leg

156

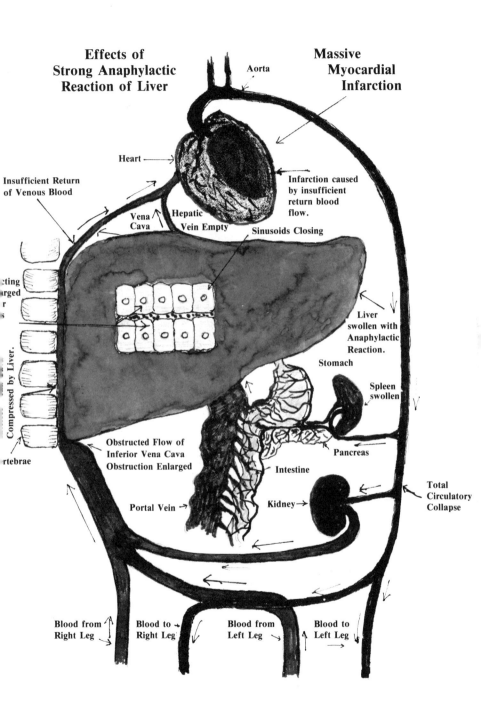

Effects of
Strong Anaphylactic
Reaction of Liver

Massive
Myocardial
Infarction

Aorta

Heart

Insufficient Return
of Venous Blood

Vena
Cava

Hepatic
Vein Empty

Infarction caused
by insufficient
return blood
flow.

Sinusoids Closing

...cting
...rged
...r
...s

Compressed by Liver.

...rtebrae

Liver
swollen with
Anaphylactic
Reaction.

Stomach

Spleen
swollen

Obstructed Flow of
Inferior Vena Cava
Obstruction Enlarged

Pancreas

Intestine

Portal Vein →

Kidney →

Total
Circulatory
Collapse

Blood from
Right Leg

Blood to →
Right Leg

Blood from
Left Leg

Blood to
Left Leg

157

Anaphylactic Liver Cell Reaction
(a)   Normal Blood Flow

Hepatic
Artery

Portal Vein

Hepatic Vein

Normal Liver Cells

Sinusoidal Canals

During Anaphylactic Reaction
(b)   Obstructed Blood Flow through Liver Canals

Blood Leaves

Hepatic Artery

Blood Enters Canals

Hepatic Vein

Portal Vein

Cyanosed Swollen Liver Cells in Anaphylaxis
Narrow or Close the Sinusoidal Canal.

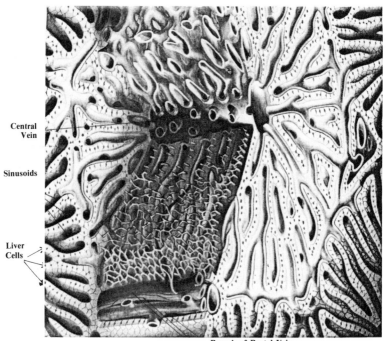

Central
Vein

Sinusoids

Liver
Cells

Sinusoids

Branch of Portal Vein
Bile Ducts
Hepatic Artery